Shoulder Arthrography

Technique, Diagnosis, and Clinical Correlation

THE LITTLE, BROWN LIBRARY OF RADIOLOGY
Herbert L. Abrams, M.D., Series Editor

Shoulder Arthrography

Technique, Diagnosis, and Clinical Correlation

Amy Beth Goldman, M.D.

Associate Professor of Radiology
Cornell University Medical College, New York City
Attending Radiologist
Hospital for Special Surgery, New York City

WITH

David M. Dines, M.D.

Clinical Instructor of Orthopaedic Surgery
Cornell University Medical College, New York City
Attending Orthopaedic Surgeon
North Shore University Hospital, Manhasset, New York
and Hospital for Special Surgery, New York City

Russell F. Warren, M.D.

Assistant Professor of Orthopaedic Surgery
Cornell University Medical College, New York City
Director of Sports Medicine and Director of Shoulder Service
Hospital for Special Surgery, New York City

FOREWORD BY R. H. FREIBERGER, M.D.

Professor of Radiology
Cornell University Medical College, New York City
Director of Radiology
Hospital for Special Surgery, New York City

LITTLE, BROWN AND COMPANY, BOSTON

Library of Congress Catalog Card No. 82-82686

ISBN 0-316-31931-7

Printed in the United States of America

HAL

WITH GRATITUDE TO THE THREE MEN
WHO HAVE SUPPORTED ME THROUGHOUT MY CAREER:
ALBERT ZIEGLER, DAVID S. GOLDMAN, M.D., AND ROBERT H. FREIBERGER, M.D.

Contents

Foreword

Combing one's hair, scratching one's back, throwing a ball, and hugging another person would not be possible were it not for the great range of motion of the shoulder. However, this facility is purchased at the price of poor bony support. The muscles and tendons that provide both stability and motion at the shoulder are therefore more subject to injury and degenerative changes causing pain and limitation of function than those of other, more stable joints. Shoulder pain is particularly annoying because it is worse when lying down than standing up and it therefore interferes with sleep.

When a patient with shoulder pain seeks medical attention, the standard roentgen examination that follows a thorough clinical exam usually consists of external and internal rotation views of the shoulder. If these reveal the amorphous calcium deposits typical of acute calcific peritendonitis, specific treatment can be offered. But when no calcium deposits are present or when the calcium deposits appear old and very dense, the shoulder arthrogram becomes a valuable diagnostic aid primarily in the detection and evaluation of rotator cuff tears. Several other conditions can also be seen, such as frozen shoulder, bicipital tendon abnormalities, capsular and articular cartilage and glenoid fibrocartilaginous rim defects that follow dislocation. The arthrogram is *the* important clinical diagnostic tool because so many of the abnormalities of the shoulder have such similar signs and symptoms that it is often difficult or impossible to arrive at a definitive diagnosis by clinical examination and routine x-ray examination alone.

It took a long time for shoulder arthrography to become the acceptable and widely used diagnostic procedure it is today. The delay in the acceptance of shoulder arthrography as a diagnostic test was for technical rather than clinical reasons. It was not until the wide distribution of image-amplified fluoroscopes with television monitoring that radiologic invasive and injection procedures could be carried out with ease in lighted rooms. Since image-amplified fluoroscopic equipment is not normally available to orthopaedic surgeons in their office practices, invasive procedures had to await a new breed of radiologists interested in and trained to perform them. At first a single and then a double contrast arthrography was practiced. By the 1960s the various factors facilitating arthrography were in place, and most orthopaedic surgeons had become familiar with the benefits of arthrography. Dr. Goldman makes a persuasive case for the advantages of double contrast arthrography. The reader who is a radiologist will recognize that the trend to double contrast examination is not unique to arthrography but is also gaining in gastrointestinal radiology.

The fully trained radiologist has to be capable of performing and interpreting shoulder arthrograms, and orthopaedic surgeons who need to know how to interpret arthrograms may wish to know how to perform them as well. This book should be helpful to both. Primarily, however, the patient benefits from arthrography; with its help the physician can arrive at a definitive diagnosis and thus a definitive therapy.

R. H. Freiberger, M.D.

Preface

Shoulder Arthrography has been written to accomplish two specific goals. The first of these is to collect the kinds of information contained in more than one thousand double contrast shoulder arthrograms performed at the Hospital for Special Surgery. The technique of double contrast shoulder arthrography is an old one that has received wide acceptance only within the past four years. It is hoped that the material presented here will demonstrate the spectrum of changes that can be identified by using the combined air-contrast study.

The second goal is to establish communication between the radiologist and the orthopaedic surgeon. *Shoulder Arthrography* will inform the radiologist about the type of information that the surgeon finds useful, and in turn, inform the surgeon about the information that is available from the shoulder arthrogram. Without good communication between the clinician and the radiologist, it is difficult to tailor the study to the individual patient, and inevitably information will be lost. It is our hope that we have written a book that will facilitate communication between, as well as be of use to, both the radiologist and the orthopaedic surgeon.

A. B. G.
D. M. D.
R. F. W.

Acknowledgments

We wish to thank the entire orthopaedic staff at the Hospital for Special Surgery for providing the case material used in this text.

We especially would like to recognize the contribution of Dr. Bernard Ghelman without whose ingenuity and originality in modifying the double contrast technique, this text would not have been possible.

The assistance of the following people must also be specifically recognized: Jill Spiller, Editorial Assistant; Patricia Boggia, with the assistance of Joyce Darwood, Secretarial Staff; Dottie Page and staff, Photography; and Hugh Thomas, medical artist.

We also would like to thank Curtis Vouwie of Little, Brown and Company for his support and advice.

Shoulder Arthrography

Technique, Diagnosis, and Clinical Correlation

1

History, Indications, Contraindications, and Complications of Shoulder Arthrography

HISTORY OF SHOULDER ARTHROGRAPHY

The technique of shoulder arthrography was first reported by Oberholzer [3], in 1933. In the majority of his early studies and those reported by Frostad [3], in 1942, air was utilized as the only contrast medium. However, in several examinations a combination of air and abrodil was used experimentally [3]. In 1939, Lindblom [10] first used the single positive contrast study. However, in the next decade, series reported by Kessel [8] and Nelson [12] emphasized the need for improvements both in injection techniques and in contrast media.

With the development of less toxic water soluble contrast materials, investigators in the late 1950s and 1960s rapidly adopted Lindblom's single positive contrast study. Series comparing the results of shoulder arthrography with surgical findings were reported by Axen [1], Kerwein et al. [7], Neviaser [13, 14], and Samilson et al. [16, 17]. These studies confirmed the usefulness of shoulder arthrography in preoperative diagnosis of rotator cuff tears [1, 7, 13, 16, 17], adhesive capsulitis [7, 14, 16, 17], biceps tendon abnormalities [7, 16, 17], and capsular changes associated with anterior dislocations [7, 16, 17]. In the late 1960s and early 1970s, the filming and injection techniques of single contrast shoulder arthrography were further refined and improved by Killoran et al. [9] and by Schneider et al. [18].

The double contrast technique of shoulder arthrography, although first reported in 1942 [3], was largely abandoned in the United States for three decades. In England, it remained the procedure of choice at the Royal National Orthopaedic Hospital in London [19] and at the Harlow Wood Orthopaedic Hospital in Nottingham [15]. In 1977, Dr. Bernard Ghelman, at the Hospital for Special Surgery, significantly improved the double contrast technique by adding upright internal and external rotation views to the filming routine.

Several published studies [2, 4, 5, 11] have confirmed that the double contrast arthrogram provides clinically useful information not obtainable from the single contrast study. First, both single and double contrast shoulder arthrograms provide an accurate means of demonstrating rotator cuff tears, but on single contrast studies the margins of the tendons are not easily visualized, and the evaluation of degenerative changes is difficult. Second, on single contrast studies, evaluation of the tendon of the long head of the biceps brachii is hampered by contrast pooling over its intracapsular insertion and by a high incidence of failure to fill the biceps tendon sheath. Third, on single contrast studies, the articular cartilages are obscured by the dense contrast material, making it difficult, even with tomography, to detect defects in the joint surfaces. Based on the superior visualization of the intra-articular structures by double contrast arthrography, and based on the fact that the double contrast study takes no more time or effort to perform than the single contrast arthrogram, the double contrast technique has become standard at the Hospital for Special Surgery.

INDICATIONS FOR DOUBLE CONTRAST SHOULDER ARTHROGRAPHY

The general indication for double contrast studies of the shoulder joint is the evaluation of structures that cannot be directly appreciated on plain films: the capsule, the articular cartilages, and the ligaments.

The shoulder joint has two tendinous structures that can be evaluated on the double contrast arthrogram: the rotator cuff and the tendon of the long head of the biceps brachii (Table 1). The rotator cuff is composed of a confluence of four tendons: the subscapularis, the supraspinatus, the infraspinatus, and the teres minor. Frequent abnormalities include traumatic tears and degenerative tears (Table 1). The rotator cuff is extra-articular and is not visualized on a normal shoulder arthrogram. It is visualized when the tendons tear and create a rent in the capsule. The origin of the tendon of the long head of the biceps brachii, unlike the rotator cuff, is intra-articular and is visualized on normal contrast studies. Common abnormalities of the biceps tendon include complete or partial ruptures, tendinitis, and medial dislocation (Table 1).

The articular cartilages of the humeral head and glenoid are also visualized on the double contrast

Table 1. *Indications for Shoulder Arthrography*

Tendon Abnormalities	Cartilage Abnormalities	Capsular Abnormalities
Rotator cuff Traumatic tears Degenerative tears Long head of the biceps brachii Tears Tendinitis Medial dislocation	Traumatic defects associated with dislocations Arthritic changes Loose bodies Secondary changes related to osteonecrosis	Adhesive capsulitis Postdislocation laxity Synovitis

shoulder arthrogram. The most common cartilage abnormalities identified on the contrast studies are post-traumatic defects that result from a previous anterior dislocation (the Hill-Sachs deformity and the Bankart deformity) (Table 1). Other cartilage abnormalities that can be identified by arthrography include arthritic changes, loose bodies, and damage due to subjacent osteonecrosis.

Lastly, the synovial-lined joint capsule is also clearly outlined, permitting the diagnosis either of a decreased capacity associated with adhesive capsulitis or of an increased capacity associated with one or more dislocations. Synovial changes associated with inflammatory or proliferative arthritides can also be visualized prior to joint space narrowing.

CONTRAINDICATIONS AND COMPLICATIONS

The two principal contraindications to shoulder arthrography are superficial skin infections and a previous severe, allergic reaction to iodinated contrast material.

In a patient with a soft tissue infection adjacent to the shoulder, an approach to the joint can be selected that avoids the area of involvement. At the Hospital for Special Surgery, an anterior approach aimed toward the midportion of the glenohumeral joint is the routine technique. However, anterolateral [20], anterosuperior [12, 13, 14], and anteroinferior [17, 18] approaches have also been described and can be used for those patients with soft tissue abnormalities. For patients who have experienced allergic reactions following the administration of contrast agents, prophylactic premedication is advisable. In individuals with a history of urticaria, Benadryl (diphenhydramine), 50 mg, is administered intramuscularly 20 minutes before the study. In patients who have experienced a cardiorespiratory collapse, the necessity of shoulder arthrography should be carefully considered. If a diagnosis is absolutely necessary, arthroscopy or a single contrast air study should be performed.

The complications of shoulder arthrography are discussed in descending order of frequency. Fortunately, most of the problems are transitory.

The most frequent clinical complaint associated with shoulder arthrography is an exacerbation of local pain beginning 2 to 4 hours after the study. Hall et al. [6] have reported the incidence of post-arthrogram pain as 74 percent; and they attribute the pain to a combination of irritation of the synovium by the positive contrast agent and to distention of the capsule following the gradual dilution of the hyperosmolar positive contrast. Both Hall and the radiologists at the Hospital for Special Surgery have noted that there is less pain following a double contrast study, probably because less positive contrast media is injected.

Syncopal reactions are associated with all invasive procedures. In over 1000 unpublished studies conducted by the authors, 12 reactions have occurred. In only one instance, did the temporary loss of consciousness interfere with the successful completion of the arthrogram. Vasovagal reactions most frequently complicate studies performed on athletic young males. Since shoulder arthrograms are most commonly done on middle-aged individuals who are likely candidates for rotator cuff tears, this problem occurs less frequently than it would in a series of knee arthrograms.

Allergic reactions to iodinated contrast material are unusual following a shoulder arthrogram. In 1075 cases performed at the Hospital for Special Surgery over a five-year period (1975–1981), only two cases of urticaria occurred. There were no major cardiorespiratory problems.

Axillary blocks have inadvertently been performed in 2 of 1075 cases. This complication most often occurs when the patient is obese and the direction of the 22-gauge needle is difficult to control. In heavy or "barrel chested" individuals, it is advisable to use a wider 20-gauge needle which, although slightly more uncomfortable for the patient, is easier to control by the examiner.

Intraosseous injections are another unusual cause of morbidity (2 of 1075 cases). This complication occurs when the tip of the needle becomes embedded between the articular cartilage and the

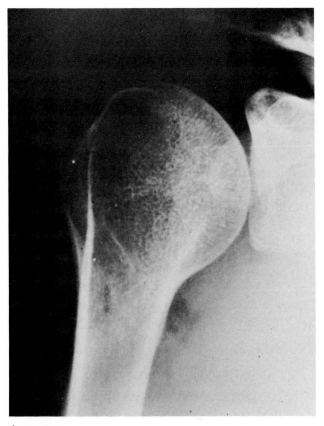

A

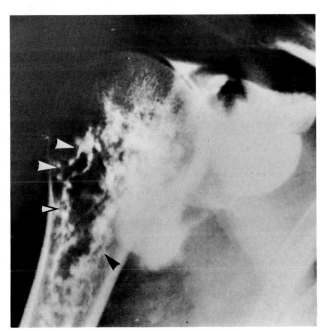

B

FIGURE 1-1. *Intraosseous injection.*
A. Preliminary external rotation view shows the humerus to be normal.
B. Postinjection internal rotation view reveals an infarct-like density in the shaft of the bone (arrows).

bone. Since part of the bevel is in the joint, the test injection may appear to confirm the intra-articular position of the needle. However, with the injection of a greater amount of contrast material, the patient experiences severe pain, and examination of the fluoroscopic image will demonstrate the presence of an osseous density that closely resembles a bone infarct (Fig. 1-1). Pain experienced during the injection of contrast agent may result either from an intraosseous injection or from adhesive capsulitis. In both instances, the shoulder should be fluoroscoped and the injection should be stopped. Fortunately, the pain from an intraosseous injection, although severe, lasts only a few hours.

Infection following a shoulder arthrogram has not occurred at the Hospital for Special Surgery. However, it is a potential danger in any study in which a needle enters a joint. Cloudy fluid, if obtained from the joint space, is always sent to the laboratory for culture and sensitivity. This precaution will eliminate the possibility that the contrast study will be blamed for cases of preexisting infection.

REFERENCES

1. Axen, O. Uber den wert der arthrographie des schultergelenkes. *Acta Radiol.* [*Diagn.*] 22:268, 1941.
2. El-Khoury, G. Y., Albright, J. P., Yousef, M. M. A., et al. Arthrotomography of the glenoid labrum. *Radiology* 131:333, 1979.
3. Fischedick, O., and Haage, H. Die Kontrast darstellung der schultergelenke. In *Encyclopedia of Medical Radiology.* Berlin: Springer, 1973. Pp. 295–304.
4. Ghelman, B., and Goldman, A. B. The double contrast shoulder arthrogram. Evaluation of rotator cuff tears. *Radiology* 124:251, 1977.
5. Goldman, A. B., and Ghelman, B. The double contrast shoulder arthrogram. Review of 158 studies. *Radiology* 127:655, 1978.
6. Hall, F. M., Rosenthal, D. I., Goldberg, R. P., et al. Morbidity from shoulder arthrography. Etiology, incidence and prevention. *A. J. R.* 139:59, 1981.
7. Kerwein, G. H., Roseberg, B., and Sneed, W. R. Arthrographic studies of the shoulder joint. *J. Bone Joint Surg.* 31(A):1267, 1957.
8. Kessel, A. W. L. Arthrography of the shoulder joint. *Proc. R. Soc. Med.* 43:418, 1950.
9. Killoran, P. J., Marcove, R. C., and Freiberger, R. H. Shoulder arthrography. *A. J. R.* 103:658, 1968.
10. Lindblom, K., and Palmer, I. Ruptures of the tendon aponeurosis of the shoulder joint. The so-

called supraspinatus ruptures. *Acta Chir. Scand.* 82:133, 1939.

11. Mink, J. H., Richardson, A., and Grant, T. T. Evaluation of glenoid labrum by double contrast shoulder arthrography. *A. J. R.* 133:883, 1979.

12. Nelson, D. H. Arthrography of the shoulder joint. *Br. J. Radiol.* 25:134, 1952.

13. Neviaser, J. S. Ruptures of the rotator cuff. *Clin. Orthop.* 3:92, 1954.

14. Neviaser, J. S. Arthrography of the shoulder joint. Study of findings in adhesive capsulitis of shoulders. *J. Bone Joint Surg.* (A):1321, 1962.

15. Preston, B. J., and Jackson, J. P. Investigation of shoulder disability by arthrography. *Clin. Radiol.* 28:259, 1977.

16. Samilson, R. L., Raphael, R. L., Post, L., et al. Arthrography of the shoulder joint. *Clin. Orthop.* 20:21, 1961.

17. Samilson, R. L., Raphael, R. L., Post, L., et al. Shoulder arthrography. *J.A.M.A.* 175:773, 1961.

18. Schneider, R., Ghelman, B., and Kaye, J. J. A simplified injection technique for shoulder arthrography. *Radiology* 114:738, 1975.

19. Stoker, D. Personal communication, 1976.

20. Tirman, R. M., Janeck, C. J., Ewsanks, R. G., et al. Shoulder arthrography: Necessary or not. Veterans Administration Hospital, Little Rock, Arkansas, 1979.

2 Anatomy of the Glenohumeral Joint

As with all arthrograms, both the performance and the interpretation depend on understanding the pertinent features of the gross anatomy.

The shoulder is a universal joint consisting of four separate articulations: the glenohumeral, the scapular-thoracic, the sternoclavicular, and the acromioclavicular. However, it is only the glenohumeral joint that can be evaluated by the shoulder arthrogram, and in this text, unless otherwise specified, the terms *shoulder* and *glenohumeral* are used synonymously.

BONE AND CARTILAGE

The humeral head articulates against a shallow glenoid fossa that covers one third of its surface. It is this osseous configuration that permits the glenohumeral joint a greater range of motion than any other joint in the body. However, by the same token, the osseous configuration provides the joint only minimal stabilization.

Both articular surfaces are covered by hyaline cartilage, but the glenoid has an additional circumferential rim or labrum that makes it more cup-shaped than can be appreciated on plain film studies (Figs. 2-1, 2-2). The labrum is composed of dense fibrous tissue combined with elastic fibers. Strands from the anterior glenoid labrum interconnect with the periosteum of the glenoid, with the hyaline cartilage of the glenoid, and with the synovial-lined joint capsule.

ADJACENT SOFT TISSUE STRUCTURES

The stability of the glenohumeral joint is largely dependent on the adjacent soft tissue structures. The scapulohumeral articulation is surrounded and reinforced by three distinct coverings, one inside the other (the joint capsule, the rotator cuff, and the subacromial-subdeltoid bursa).

Joint Capsule

Closest to the bone and cartilage is the synovial-lined joint capsule (Fig. 2-3). The capsule is a loose, fibrous structure having approximately twice the surface area of the humeral head. Distally, it attaches to the humerus adjacent to the greater tuberosity and then crosses medially at the

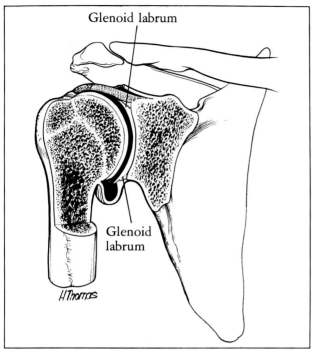

FIGURE 2-2. *Diagram of the glenoid labrum.*
The glenoid is seen in profile, as it would be on a contrast arthrogram. The upper and lower corners are wider than the center.

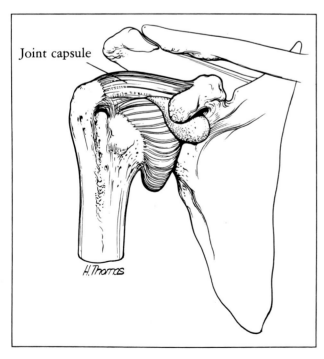

FIGURE 2-3. *Diagram of the joint capsule demonstrating the insertion along the humeral neck, the subscapularis bursa, and axillary recess.*

level of the anatomic neck. Proximally, the posterior margin of the capsule inserts on the neck of the scapula and the anterior margin of the capsule inserts into the glenoid labrum and its underlying bone. The proximal capsule attachment is intimately associated with and actually incorporated into the glenoid labrum. At surgical exploration the capsule and labrum cannot be identified as separate structures. Localized areas of capsular thickening are referred to as the superior, inferior, and middle glenohumeral ligaments.

The joint capsule has two normal recesses: (1) the axillary recess that hangs between the scapula and humerus and provides the necessary redundancy for elevation of the arm, and (2) the subscapularis bursa that lies immediately below the coracoid process. Although it is a separate pocket, the subscapularis bursa has a consistent communication with the capsule.

Rotator Cuff

Surrounding the synovial-lined joint capsule (and in some areas actually incorporated into it) is a strong reinforcing sheath composed of the tendons of the rotator cuff: the supraspinatus, the infraspinatus, the teres minor, and the subscapularis (Figs. 2-4, 2-5).

The supraspinatus muscle originates on the supraspinous portion of the scapula and inserts on the superior aspect of the greater tuberosity (Fig. 2-5). During its course it is compressed tightly against the acromioclavicular joint and the coracoacromial ligament. The infraspinatus muscle arises from the infraspinous portion of the scapula and inserts on the posterior aspect of the greater tuberosity. The teres minor, a less important part of the rotator cuff than the supraspinatus, originates on the axillary border of the scapular and attaches to the inferior surface of the greater tuberosity. The last of the four tendons is the subscapularis, which takes its origin from the subscapularis fossa and forms the anterior aspect of the rotator cuff. Unlike the supraspinatus, infraspinatus, and teres minor tendons, the subscapularis inserts on the lesser tuberosity, and also unlike the three other tendons, it is not only part of the rotator cuff, but also acts as a significant internal rotator of the shoulder.

As a whole, the tendinous rotator cuff occupies almost the entire space between the humeral head and the acromion process (as seen on the plain

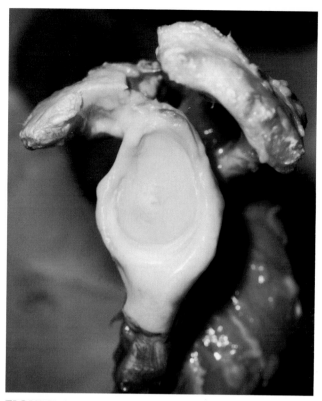

FIGURE 2-1. *Dissection of the glenoid labrum.*
The cavity of the glenoid is seen en face. The labrum, which forms its rim, is interconnected with the hyalin cartilage of the glenoid and with the periosteum of the scapula.

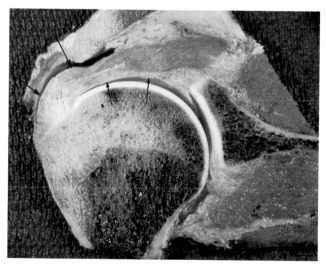

FIGURE 2-4. *Dissection of the rotator cuff.*
Small arrows indicate the joint capsule lining its inner surface; large arrows indicate the subacromial-subdeltoid bursa covering its outer surface.

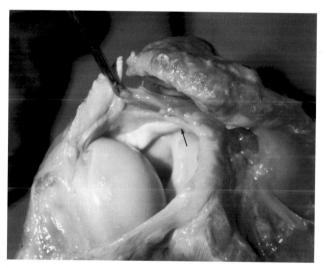

FIGURE 2-7. *Dissection of the intra-articular portion of the tendon of the long head of the biceps brachii.*
The insertion of this tendon, just above the glenoid labrum, is marked by an arrow.

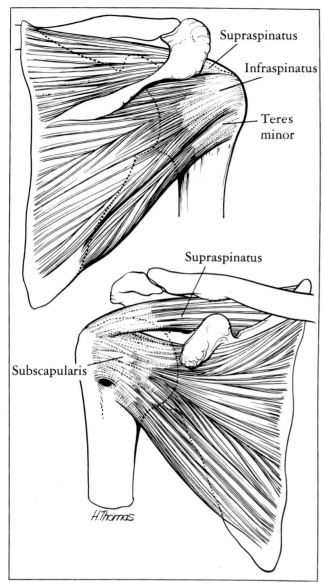

Supraspinatus

Infraspinatus

Teres minor

Supraspinatus

Subscapularis

H.Thomas

FIGURE 2-5. *Diagram of the anterior and posterior surfaces of the rotator cuff.*

films). It envelops the humeral head and both fixes the humeral head within the glenoid and causes the humeral head to descend as the humerus is abducted by the deltoid. The interaction between the deltoid and the rotator cuff is complex, but essentially the rotator cuff provides the fulcrum for the deltoid muscle. In turn, the deltoid is the prime abductor of the arm. The power of the deltoid, therefore, depends on the integrity of the rotator cuff.

Subacromial-Subdeltoid Bursa

Outside of the rotator cuff is the third, thin, soft tissue covering on the anterior surface of the glenohumeral joint. It is composed of the subacromial bursa, which lies immediately below the osseous acromion process, and the subdeltoid bursa, which lies under the deltoid muscle (Fig. 2-6). In some individuals, the subcoracoid bursa also forms a part of the bursal sac. The subacromial-subdeltoid bursae are actually a single structure with two names. For the purpose of this text, they will be referred to as a single, connected bursa with a hyphenated name. The only way in which the subacromial and subdeltoid bursa can communicate with the joint capsule is if there is a complete interruption of the intervening rotator cuff.

Coracoacromial Ligament

The humeral head and its three soft tissue integuments are, in turn, covered by the coracoacromial arch. Composed of the acromion, the coracoid, and the fixed angular coracoacromial ligament, the coracoacromial arch provides a roof for the glenohumeral joint (Fig. 2-6). The exact function of the coracoacromial ligament is not understood. However, due to its close relationship to the humeral head, any irregularity of the adjacent bone will cause an impedance to abduction, which may lead to friction, irritation, and ultimately to inflammation of the bursa and degeneration of the rotator cuff. The supraspinatus, due to its proximity to the coracoacromial arch, is particularly vulnerable.

TENDON OF THE LONG HEAD OF THE BICEPS

The tendon of the long head of the biceps inserts above the superior glenoid labrum. From its insertion to the bicipital groove, it is an intra-articular

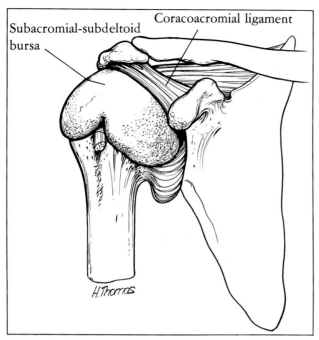

FIGURE 2-6. *Diagram of the subacromial-subdeltoid bursa, which is superficial to the anterior aspect of the rotator cuff.*

The coracoacromial ligament is also shown. This ligament, in combination with the osseous acromion and coracoid, form the roof of the glenohumeral joint.

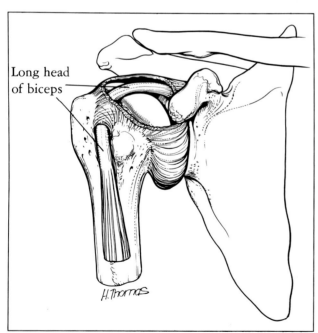

FIGURE 2-8. *Diagram of the tendon of the long head of the biceps brachii.*

From its insertion on the superior glenoid labrum to the bicipital groove, the tendon is within the capsule. Within the bicipital groove and below it, the tendon remains covered by a capsular reflection called the tendon sheath.

structure (Figs. 2-7, 2-8). Between the tuberosities and for a variable distance below them, the tendon remains covered by a synovial-lined capsular reflection (Figs. 2-7, 2-8). Therefore both the intracapsular and intrasheath portions of the biceps tendon should be visualized on a normal shoulder arthrogram.

The walls of the bicipital groove are the greater and lesser tuberosities that face anterolaterally approximately 15° to the humeral axis. The roof of the groove is formed by a combination of the rotator cuff, the transverse humeral ligament, the acromioclavicular joint, and the undersurface of the acromion. Damage to any of these structures can also affect the tendon of the long head of the biceps.

During elevation of the arm, the groove slides approximately one to one and one-half inches along the tendon. Electromyogram studies indicate that the tendon is active in abduction, external rotation, and occasionally, in forward flexion. It is believed that the tendon of the long head of the biceps prevents superior migration of the humeral head.

SUGGESTED READING

Bateman, J. E. *The Shoulder and Neck* (2nd ed.). Philadelphia: Saunders, 1978. Pp. 47–116.

Bechtol, C. O. Biomechanics of the shoulder. *Clin. Orthop.* 146:37, 1980.

DePalma, A. I. Surgical anatomy of the acromioclavicular and sternoclavicular joints. *Surg. Clin. North Am.* 43:1541, 1963.

Grant, J. E. B. The Upper Limb. In J. E. Anderson (ed.), *Grant's Atlas of Anatomy* (7th ed.). Baltimore: Williams & Wilkins, 1978. Pp. 6-15–6-49A.

Neer, C. S., II, and Rockwood, C. A., Jr. Fractures and Dislocations of the Shoulder. In C. A. Rockwood, Jr. and D. P. Green (eds.), *Fractures*. Philadelphia: Lippincott, 1975. Pp. 586–587.

Sobatta, J., and Figge, F. H. *Atlas of Human Anatomy* (9th ed.). New York: Hafner, 1974. Pp. 109–111.

3

Technique

PRELIMINARY FILMS

Four routine studies are obtained prior to the shoulder arthrogram: the internal rotation view, the external rotation view, the axillary view, and the bicipital groove view. For patients with a history of either dislocation or subluxation of the glenohumeral joint, three films are added to this routine. As with the four standard preliminary views, the extra studies are obtained both before and after the injection of contrast material. Specifically, the additional views are the West Point prone axillary view, the Stryker or "notch" view, and the Didiee view. These additional studies are referred to as the "instability series," and they demonstrate various profiles of the humerus and glenoid and allow greater visualization of the articular surfaces of both structures.

The internal rotation view is filmed with the patient's back flat against the examination table and the arm internally rotated as far as possible. The central beam of the x-ray tube is centered on the humeral head and is angled 15° toward the feet to open up the soft tissue space between the humerus and the acromion process (Fig. 3-1A). On an ideal internal rotation view, the humerus should be sufficiently rotated so that on the medial aspect the lesser tuberosity is seen in profile and the lateral side is perfectly smooth and spherical (Fig. 3-1B).

For the external rotation view, the shoulder is filmed in a 15° to 25° posterior oblique position (Fig. 3-2A). In most individuals, this degree of obliquity will provide a tangential view of the glenohumeral joint space. On an adequate external rotation view, both tuberosities are seen in profile, forming a portion of the lateral margin of the humeral head (Fig. 3-2B).

The bicipital groove view can be filmed with the patient standing, sitting, or supine. The cassette is held perpendicular to the superior surface of the humerus, and the shoulder is positioned in maximal internal rotation. The central beam is directed parallel to the long axis of the humerus (Fig. 3-3A). On an adequate bicipital groove view, the humeral head is spherical and the tuberosities and groove appear along its superior articular surface (Fig. 3-3B).

For the routine axillary view at the Hospital for Special Surgery, the patient is supine on the x-ray

12

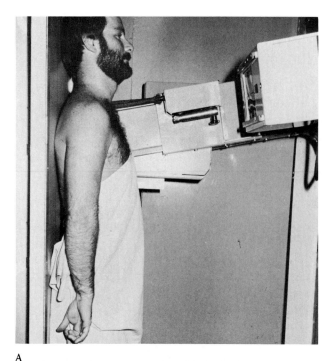

A

B

FIGURE 3-1. *Normal internal rotation view.*

A. Patient stands with back flat against the x-ray table and arm internally rotated. The central beam is angled 15° toward the feet.

B. Normal internal rotation view with the lesser tuberosity (arrow) forming part of the medial profile of the humeral head. The lateral aspect of the humeral head is smooth and spherical.

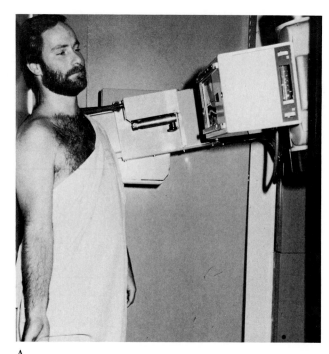

A

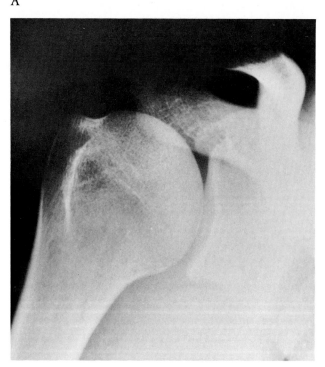

B

FIGURE 3-2. *Normal external rotation view.*

A. Patient is positioned in a 25° posterior oblique to view the joint in tangent. The central beam is angled 15° toward the feet.

B. Normal obliqued external rotation view with the glenoid seen in tangent and the tuberosities forming part of the lateral profile of the humeral head.

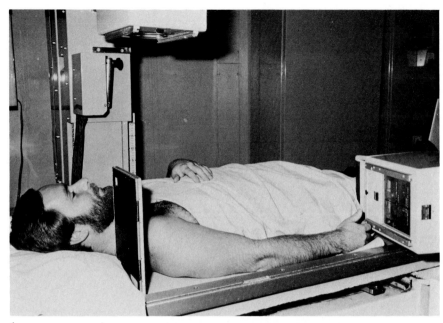

A

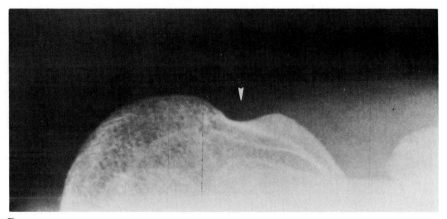

B

FIGURE 3-3. *Normal bicipital groove view.*
A. Shoulder is in maximal internal rotation and the
    central beam is parallel to the long axis of humerus.
B. The normal bicipital groove view reveals the
    tuberosities en face along the superior-anterior sur-
    faces of the humeral head. The bicipital groove lies
    between the tuberosities (arrow).

14

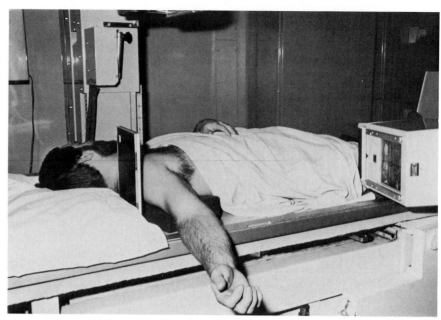

A

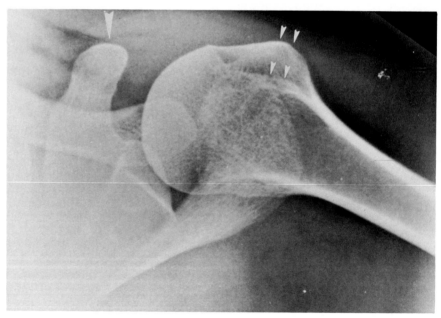

B

FIGURE 3-4. *Normal supine axillary view.*

A. The patient is positioned with the arm abducted
   90° to the body. The shoulder is externally rotated.
   The central beam is directed into the axilla.

B. The normal supine axillary view shows the
   glenohumeral joint in tangent. The coracoid process (large arrow) and the tuberosities (small arrows) mark the anterior surface of the shoulder. The
   acromioclavicular joint is superimposed on the center of the humeral head.

table. The arm is abducted 90° to the body, and the shoulder is held in external rotation with the central beam directed into the axilla (Fig. 3-4A). The supine axillary view provides an excellent means of viewing the glenohumeral joint in tangent and of seeing the bicipital groove in profile with both tuberosities visualized along the anterior aspect of the humeral head. On an adequate supine axillary view, the acromioclavicular joint should be superimposed on the center of the humeral head (Fig. 3-4B).

In patients with a history of dislocation or instability of the glenohumeral joint, the three instability studies are also obtained. These additional views can occasionally identify a small compression fracture or a small area of heterotopic ossification that is not seen on standard views (Figs. 3-5, 3-6). The first of the instability series is the West Point prone axillary view, described by Rokous et al. [3] (Fig. 3-5A). The patient is prone on the examination table with the arm abducted 90° and rotated so that its anterior surface faces upward (Fig. 3-5A). The film is then placed against the anterior surface of the shoulder (Fig. 3-5A). The central beam is angled 25° medially and 25° cephalad (Fig. 3-5A). The West Point prone axillary view provides good visualization of the anteroinferior articular surface of the glenoid and the smooth spherical posterior aspect of the humeral head (Figs. 3-5B, 3-6).

The second view of the instability series is the Stryker or notch view. The patient is turned supine on the examination table and the arm is elevated so the hand rests on top of the patient's head. The central ray is angled 10° toward the head and parallels the shaft of the humerus (Fig. 3-5C). On this view, the lesser tuberosity is seen in profile along the medial aspect of the humeral head. The greater tuberosity is superimposed on the humeral head and the posterior surface of the humerus is smooth and spherical. This view provides an excellent view of the posterolateral surface of the humeral head (Figs. 3-5D, 3-6D).

The third study is the Didiee view. The patient is prone on the x-ray table with the arm abducted and the hand placed on the iliac crest. The film is below the shoulder and the central beam is angled 45° downward and directed along the long axis of the humerus (Fig. 3-5E). This study is used to demonstrate posterolateral defects in the humeral head, and heterotopic ossification forming along the inferior surface of the glenoid (Figs. 3-5F, 3-

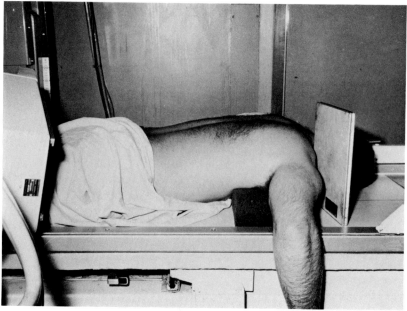

A

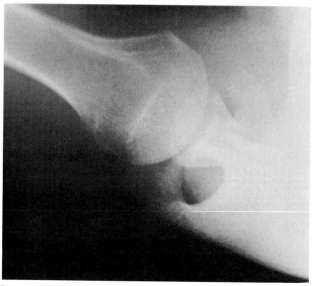

B

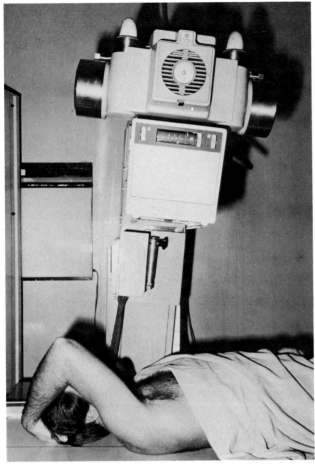

C

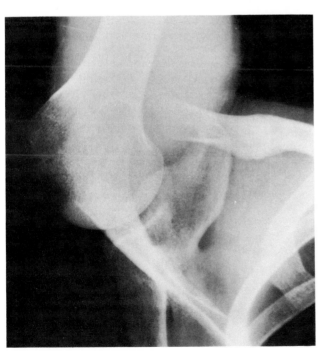

D

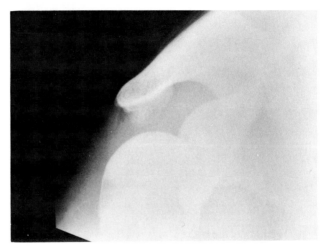

E

F

FIGURE 3-5. *Normal instability series.*

A. The prone axillary view is filmed with the arm abducted 90°. The central beam is directed at the axilla and is angled 25° medially and 25° cephalad.

B. The prone axillary view demonstrates the anterior glenoid labrum and the smooth spherical posterior aspect of the humeral head.

C. The Stryker view is filmed with the patient supine on the x-ray table and the arm elevated with the hand resting on top of the head. The central beam parallels the shaft of the humerus and is angled 10° cephalad.

D. The normal Stryker view demonstrates the rounded configuration of the posterior humeral head.

E. The Didiee view is obtained with the patient prone and the arm abducted. The hand is placed on the iliac crest. The central beam is angled 45° caudad and directed along the shaft of the humerus.

F. The normal Didiee view shows both the posterior humeral head and inferior glenoid to advantage.

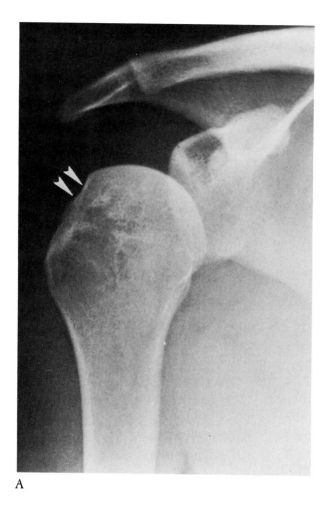

A

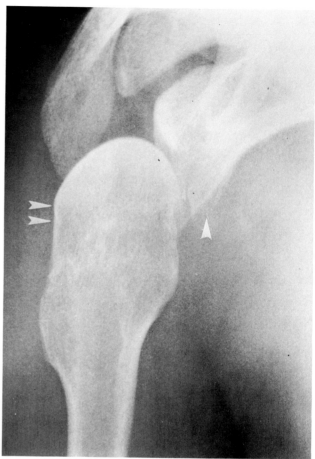

B

FIGURE 3-6. *Positive instability series.*

A. The internal rotation view shows flattening of the superior lateral aspect of the humeral head or the Hill-Sachs deformity (large arrows).

B. The obliqued external rotation view shows loss of the normal inferior cortex of the glenoid labrum or the Bankart deformity (small arrows).

C. The prone axillary view confirms the presence of the Bankart defect in the anterior glenoid labrum (small arrows) and shows its extent. Small fracture fragments or areas of heterotopic ossification are also demonstrated near the damaged glenoid. The flattening of the posterior humeral head is also shown to advantage (large arrow).

D. The Stryker view shows the Hill-Sachs defect (large arrows).

E. The Didiee view shows the Hill-Sachs defect (large arrows) and also demonstrates the glenoid defect (small arrow).

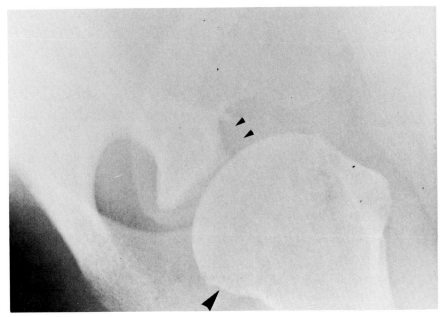

C

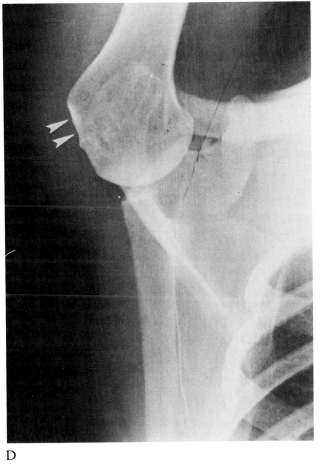

D

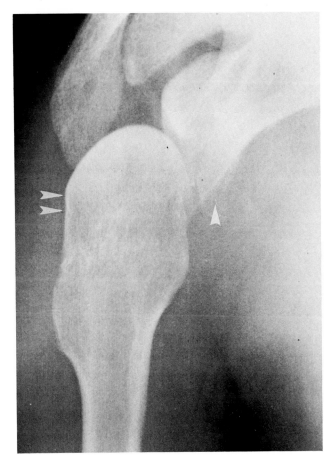

E

20

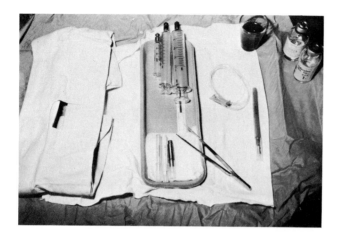

FIGURE 3-7. *Standard arthrogram tray.*
Contains a 2½-cc syringe for local anesthesia, a 10-cc
syringe for positive contrast agent, and a 20-cc syringe
for room air. A 22-gauge spinal needle and long
venotubing are added to the set.

6E). The Stryker and Didiee views are performed
using the technique described in Moseley's text on
shoulder lesions [2].

ARTHROGRAM TRAY

The standard arthrogram tray used at the Hospital
for Special Surgery includes three syringes: a 2½-
cc syringe for local anesthesia, a 10-cc syringe for
positive contrast, and a 20-cc syringe for room air
(Fig. 3-7). Also included are a glass cup for Betadine (povidone-iodine) solution, gauze sponges
to apply the disinfectant, and a sterile drape with a
central hole for covering the shoulder. There is a
selection of four needles on the tray: a 25-gauge
skin needle, a 20-gauge 1½-inch needle, an 18-
gauge 1½-inch needle, and a 16-gauge 1½-inch
needle. For a shoulder arthrogram, a 22-gauge 3½-
inch spinal needle and long venotubing must be
added to the standard set. Lidocaine, Renografin-
60 (diatrizoate meglumine and diatrizoate so-
dium), and Betadine are available on a side table.

INJECTION TECHNIQUE

The patient lies supine on the x-ray table with the
arm mildly abducted (Fig. 3-8A). The shoulder can
be positioned in either a neutral position or in mild
external rotation. As described by Schneider et al.
[4], obliquing the patient to view the joint in tangent is not advisable because it rotates the fibrous
labrum of the glenoid over the apparent joint
space and the needle meets an obstruction.

Under fluoroscopic control, a lead marker is adjusted until it is directly over the center of the
glenohumeral joint (Fig. 3-8B). This point is then
marked on the skin as the site of injection. The
center of the shoulder joint is not the widest portion of the joint space, but it is considered to be
the optimum site for the injection of contrast material. If the needle is aimed at the superior surface
of the glenohumeral joint, minimal leakage of contrast material may be misinterpreted as a rotator
cuff tear. If the needle is aimed too low, it is possible to pass through the axillary recess and miss the
joint entirely or to inadvertently administer an axillary block with lidocaine.

After the center of the glenohumeral joint is
identified and the skin is marked, the examiner
puts on sterile gloves. An assistant fills the glass
cup with a Betadine solution and the examiner

cleans both the shoulder and axilla with the disinfectant. The shoulder is then covered with a sterile drape (Fig. 3-8C). The 2½-cc syringe is filled with a small amount of 1% lidocaine. The 10-cc syringe is filled with 10 cc of Renografin-60 (only 3 to 4 cc of Renografin will be injected into the shoulder, but a larger amount is necessary since the injection is done through venotubing), and the 20-cc syringe is filled with 10 cc of room air. The 16-gauge 1½-inch needle can rapidly fill the syringes.

Following the administration of local anesthesia, the 22-gauge spinal needle is held perpendicular to the skin and passed straight down toward the cartilage space. The glenohumeral joint is quite deep (Fig. 3-8D), and after checking the position of the needle under the skin, it is advisable to advance the needle rapidly downward. If the needle touches an obstruction before it is halfway into the shoulder, the tip is probably touching the anterior aspect of the humeral head and is not in the joint. In such instances, the position of the needle should be checked under fluoroscopy and the needle redirected toward the joint. When the tip of the 22-gauge spinal needle enters the joint space, there is no palpable sensation experienced by the examiner. However, on the fluoroscopic screen, the flexible 22-gauge needle gently curves around the surface of the humeral head (Fig. 3-8E). Aspiration can be attempted at this time, but it is rare to obtain synovial fluid from the shoulder joint. The venotubing is then attached to the needle and under fluoroscopic control a test injection is performed using a small amount of positive contrast material (Fig. 3-8F). If the needle is intra-articular, the contrast material flows freely away from the needle tip and around the humeral head, across the humeral neck, or into the subscapularis bursa (Fig. 3-8G). Since contrast may flow in any of these three directions, the entire shoulder, including the coracoid process, should be visible on the fluoroscopic screen. If the needle tip is subcutaneous and not within the joint, contrast material remains pooled at the tip (Fig. 3-8H). The needle must be advanced downward. If no contrast flows through the needle, it usually indicates that the tip is too far into the joint and is stuck in the posterior glenoid labrum. In this instance, the lidocaine syringe should be reattached and the needle slightly withdrawn until the local anesthesia flows freely. The test injection can then be reattempted. Additional techniques to confirm the position of the needle

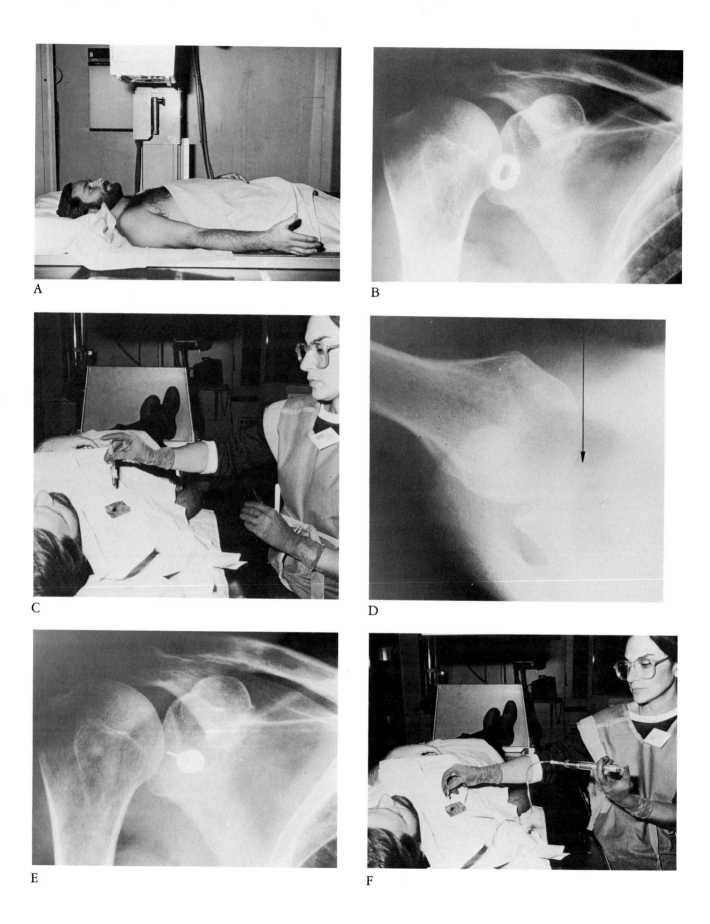

A

B

C

D

E

F

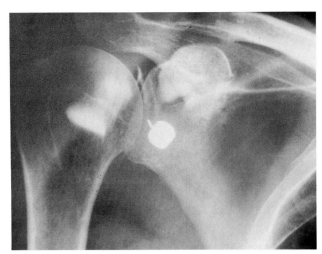

G

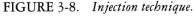

H

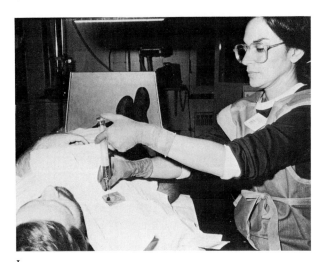

I

FIGURE 3-8. *Injection technique.*

A. The patient is placed supine on the x-ray table with the arm mildly abducted. The thumb points upward to remind him not to rotate the shoulder during the procedure.

B. Under fluoroscopic control, a lead marker is adjusted until it is directly over the center of the glenohumeral joint, and this point is marked on the skin as the site of injection.

C. After a sterile preparation of the shoulder and axilla, local anesthesia is administered. The 22-gauge 3½-inch spinal needle is held perpendicular to the skin and directed straight down.

D. An arrow superimposed on a supine axillary view demonstrates the long distance from the skin to the glenohumeral joint.

E. When the thin 22-gauge needle enters the joint, its tip curves slightly.

F. A test injection is performed through venotubing and observed on the fluoroscopic screen.

G. A successful test injection shows that the positive contrast flows rapidly away from the tip of the needle and extends across the neck around the humeral head or into the subscapularis bursa.

H. A subcutaneous injection with contrast pooling at the tip of the needle.

I. Air is injected only after the test injection with positive contrast demonstrates the needle to be intra-articular, and after 4 cc of positive contrast have been introduced. The total amount injected is 4 cc of Renografin-60 and 10 cc of room air.

prior to injection of contrast material have been described by Dalinka [1] and Wills and Diznoff [5]. Although not absolutely necessary, these methods of localization using metallic grids [1] or observing the lidocaine level in the needle [5] may be of aid to some individuals.

Following the successful placement of the needle, Renografin-60, 4 cc, is injected. The venotubing is removed and the air syringe attached to the needle (Fig. 3-8I). About 10 cc of room air is pushed into the joint and the needle is removed. For a single contrast study, Renografin-60, 12 to 15 cc, is injected instead of the air-contrast combination.

FILMING

Immediately following the injection of contrast, six routine studies are obtained for the standard double contrast shoulder arthrogram: internal and external rotation views with soft tissue technique, internal and external rotation views with overpenetrated technique, a supine axillary view, and a bicipital groove view.

The internal and external rotation views are filmed with the patient standing and the beam angled 15° toward the feet, to separate the area of the rotator cuff away from the osseous acromion process (see Figs. 3-1, 3-2). If possible, the patient is asked to hold a five-pound sand bag to produce distraction on the glenohumeral joint. Both the internal and external rotation views are filmed twice, once with the soft tissue technique for optimum visualization of the rotator cuff and the tendon of the long head of the biceps, and once with overpenetrated technique to visualize the articular cartilages and the glenoid labrum (Fig. 3-9). As with the preliminary studies, the internal rotation view is best filmed with the shoulder in a straight antero-posterior position with the patient's back flat against the x-ray table, while the external rotation view is best filmed with the patient rotated 25° posteriorly relative to the x-ray table to view the joint in tangent (Fig. 3-9). The internal and external rotation views are most accurately filmed under fluoroscopic control to determine the optimum position of the beam for visualization of the articular cartilages and the rotator cuff. If standard fluoroscopy is unavailable, adequate studies can still be obtained by estimating these factors.

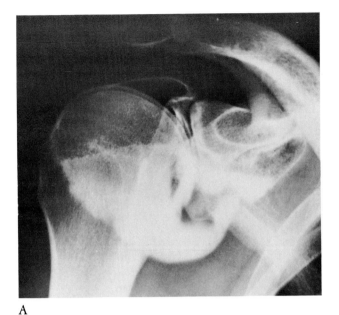

A

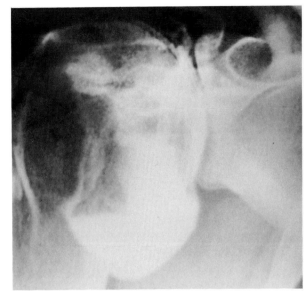

B

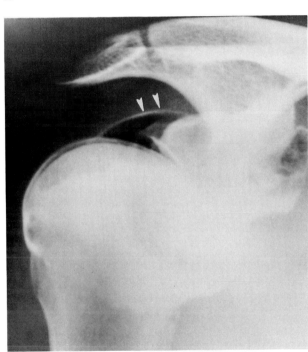

C

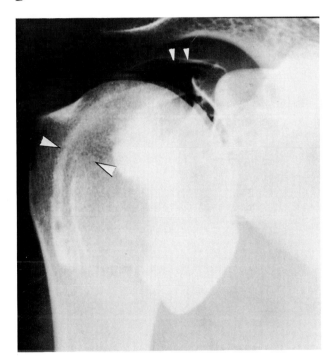

D

FIGURE 3-9.   *Routine standing views.*

A, B. Overpenetrated internal and external rotation
        views are obtained to visualize the articular
        cartilages.

C, D. Underpenetrated internal and external rotation
        views are obtained to demonstrate the inferior
        surface of the rotator cuff (small arrows) and the
        tendon of the long head of the biceps brachii
        (large arrows).

Following the standing internal and external rotation views, the patient is returned to the supine position for the axillary and bicipital groove views.

In patients with a history of dislocation or subluxation, both the injection and filming techniques are modified. First, because filming must take longer and fine detail must be apparent, a small amount of epinephrine, 1:1000 (⅓ cc), is added to the positive contrast material to delay dilution and reabsorption. Second, in cases of unstable shoulders, the amount of positive contrast material injected should be reduced by approximately 1 cc to facilitate the visualization of the bottom of the articular cartilage of the glenoid. If too much contrast is inadvertently injected, the following maneuvers can be attempted to salvage the study, particularly the tangential views of the joint.

1. An external rotation view can be obtained with the arm abducted to spread out the contrast that fills the axillary recess.
2. An external rotation view can be obtained with extreme caudad angulation of the central beam to project the contrast filled axillary recess below the cartilage.
3. An external rotation view can be attempted with the patient in Trendelenburg's position to move the excess contrast material to the top of the joint.
4. Lastly, if plain films fail, tomograms can be obtained with the humerus abducted 90°.

The third modification of the shoulder arthrogram for individuals with unstable shoulders are the additional views: the West Point prone axillary view described by Rokous [3] and the Stryker and Didiee views modified from the technique described in Moseley's text [4]. These extra studies provide more extensive visualization of the articular surfaces of the humerus and glenoid and are referred to at the Hospital for Special Surgery as the "instability series."

Regardless of the indication for the shoulder arthrogram, if the initial studies are negative, the patient is asked to exercise the shoulder and the routine films are repeated.

The filming routine for a single contrast arthrogram significantly differs from that of the double contrast study. The internal rotation, the external rotation, the axillary, and the bicipital groove views are all obtained with the patient supine. Since the margins of the articular cartilages are obscured by the dense positive contrast material, evaluation of small post-traumatic defects or early arthritic abnormalities is difficult. Additional detail may be obtained by adding tomographic studies. As with the double contrast technique, if the original studies are negative, the shoulder is exercised and the films are repeated.

REFERENCES

1. Dalinka, M. K. A simple aid to the performance of shoulder arthrography. *A. J. R.* 129:942, 1977.
2. Moseley, H. F. *Shoulder Lesions* (3rd ed.). Baltimore: Williams & Wilkins, 1969. Pp. 37–50.
3. Rokous, J. H., Feagin, J. A., and Abbott, H. G. Modified axillary view: A useful adjunct in the diagnosis of recurrent instability of the shoulder. *Clin. Orthop.* 82:84, 1972.
4. Schneider, R., Ghelman, B., and Kaye, J. J. A simplified injection technique for shoulder arthrography. *Radiology* 114:738, 1975.
5. Wills, J. S., and Diznoff, S. B. A modified technique for needle localization in arthrography of the shoulder. *Radiology* 128:830, 1978.

SUGGESTED READING

Ghelman, B., and Goldman, A. B. The double contrast shoulder arthrogram: Evaluation of rotator cuff tears. *Radiology* 124:251, 1977.

Goldman, A. B., and Ghelman, B. The double contrast shoulder arthrogram: A review of 158 cases. *Radiology* 127:655, 1978.

Kaye, J. J., and Goldman, A. B. Shoulder Arthrography. In R. H. Freiberger and J. J. Kaye (Eds.), *Arthrography*. New York: Appleton-Century-Crofts, 1979. Pp. 137–188.

Killoran, P. J., Marcove, R. C., and Freiberger, R. H. Shoulder arthrography. *A.J.R.* 103:658, 1968.

4 The Normal Shoulder Arthrogram

THE NORMAL DOUBLE CONTRAST ARTHROGRAM

Standing Internal and External Rotation Views

The air- and contrast-filled capsule has a sharp, smooth margin (Fig. 4-1A–D). Laterally, it inserts on the humeral head proximal to the greater tuberosity and then crosses the humeral neck in an oblique line. Medially, the capsule attaches to the osseous rim of the glenoid and the neck of the scapula; it is subjacent to and intimately associated with the glenoid labrum. The entire glenoid labrum is intracapsular, and contrast normally outlines its concave lateral articular surface, the superior surface of the superior glenoid labrum, and the inferior surface of the inferior glenoid labrum (Figs. 4-1 to 4-5). On the standing films, the superior aspect of the capsule, which can also be considered the bottom of the rotator cuff, is coated by contrast and outlined by air (Fig. 4-1A–D). It begins above the superior glenoid labrum and crosses the joint space. Because of the adjacent air within the joint, the capsule is seen as a distinct line. As the capsule passes laterally over the superior articular cartilage of the humeral head, its outline becomes so closely applied to the adjacent cartilage that it is indistinguishable as a separate shadow (Fig. 4-1A–D). No air or contrast should be seen above the line of the capsular roof medially or above the articular cartilage of the humeral head laterally (Fig. 4-1A–D). The inferior aspect of the joint capsule is referred to as the *axillary recess* (Figs. 4-1A–D; 4-2). It is normally a redundant area and hangs as a pouch between the humeral head and scapula. The axillary recess provides the necessary capsular laxity to permit elevation of the arm (Fig. 4-2). Therefore, on films obtained with the arm in abduction, the axillary recess is stretched out and not seen as a separate recess (Fig. 4-2). The shoulder joint capsule also has a second recess, referred to as the *subscapularis bursa* (Fig. 4-1A–D). It lies immediately below the coracoid process and gives the medial aspect of the capsule a reversed "3" configuration (Figs. 4-1A–D; 4-2).

On the overpenetrated standing external rotation view with the shoulder obliqued 25° posteriorly, the glenoid labrum is seen in profile (Figs. 4-1B, 4-2, 4-3, 4-4). It is outlined by a thin line of

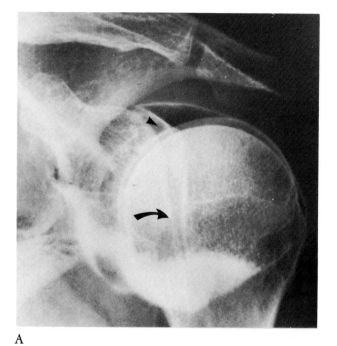

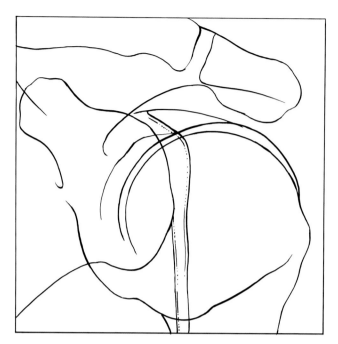

A

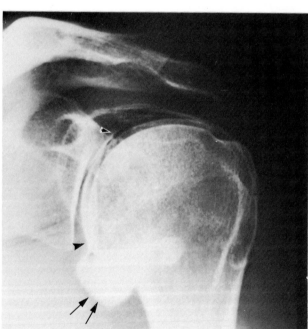

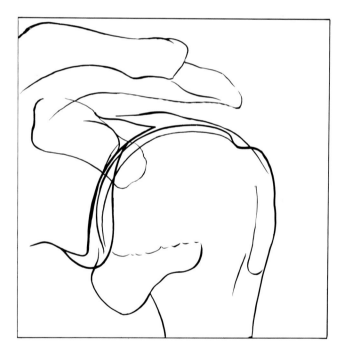

B

FIGURE 4-1. *Normal double contrast shoulder arthrogram: six pre-exercise views. Overpenetrated studies demonstrate cartilaginous detail. Underpenetrated studies show ligamentous structures.*

Small black arrowheads mark glenoid labrum. Large white arrowheads point to the top of the joint capsule, which is also the bottom of the rotator cuff. Small black arrows mark the axillary recess. The hollow black arrows show the subscapularis bursa. Curved black arrows mark the tendon of the long head of the biceps. Selected films are repeated after exercise of shoulder.

A, B. Overpenetrated standing internal and external rotation views.

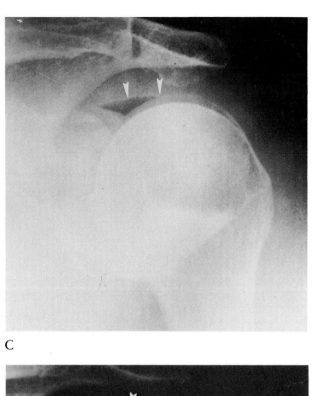
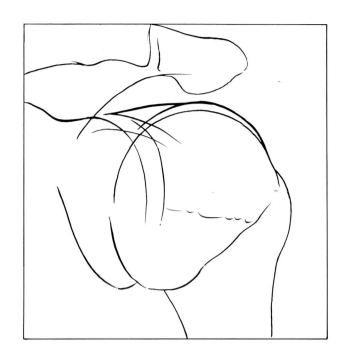

C

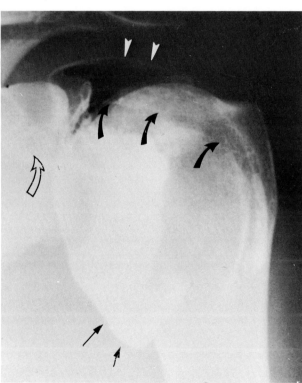
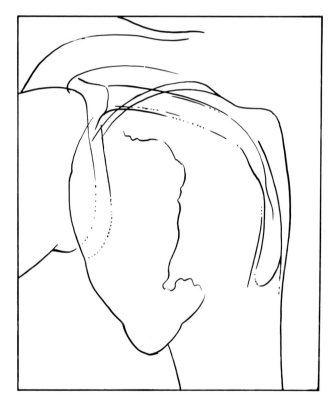

D

FIGURE 4-1. *(Continued)*
C, D. Underpenetrated standing internal and external
rotation views.

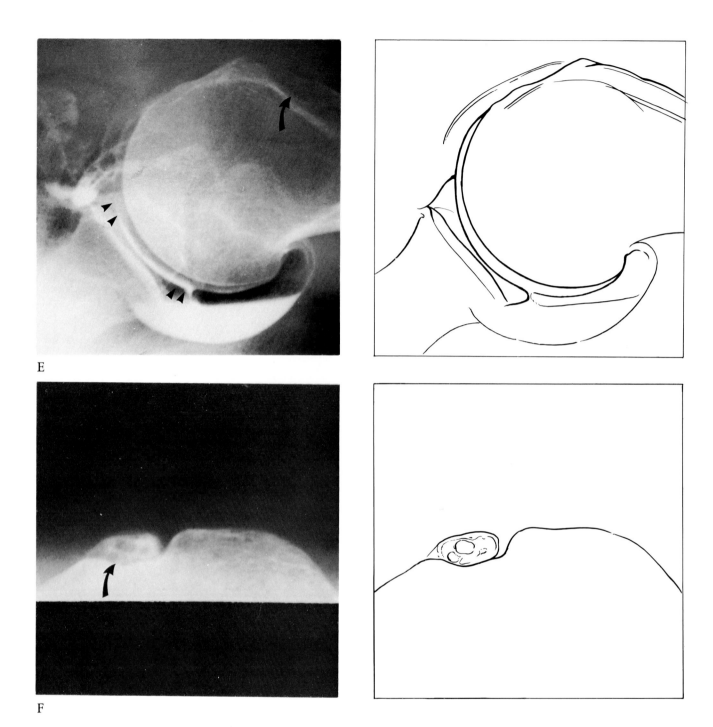

E

F

FIGURE 4-1. *(Continued)*
E. Supine axillary view.
F. Bicipital groove view.

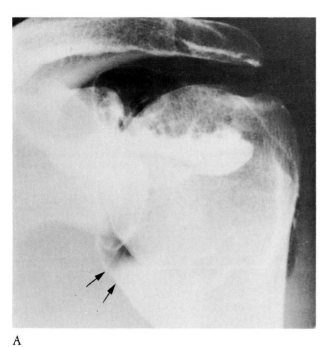

A

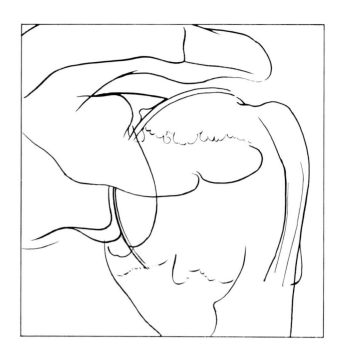

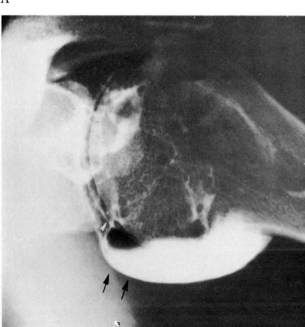

B

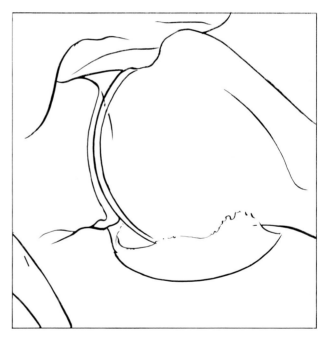

FIGURE 4-2.   *Standing external rotation views.*
A. The routine study, obtained with the patient's arm
   at his side, shows excessive contrast in the axillary
   recess (small black arrows).
B. Repeat external rotation view with the patient's arm
   elevated stretches out the axillary recess (small
   black arrows) and demonstrates the inferior glenoid
   labrum (small white arrowhead).

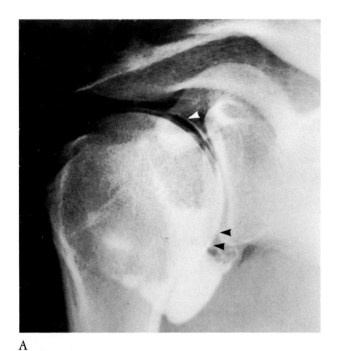

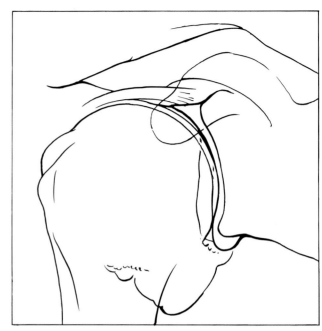

A

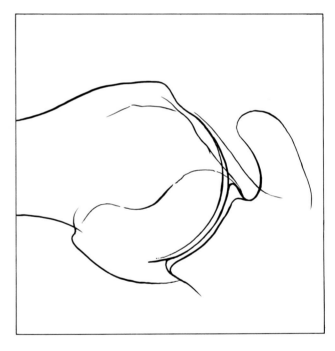

B

FIGURE 4-3. *Normal anterior glenoid labrum (small arrowheads).*

A. Overpenetrated standing external rotation view with the shoulder obliqued 25° posteriorly.

B. Supine axillary view with most of the contrast pooled in the posterior recess of the joint.

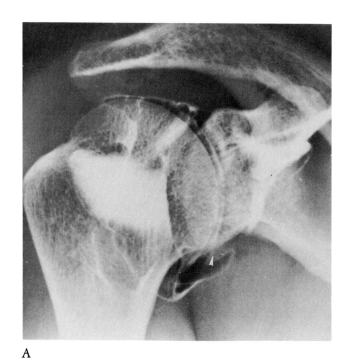
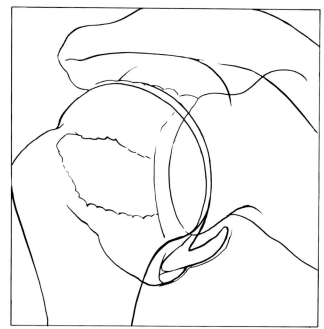

A

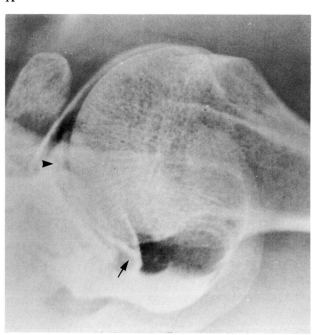
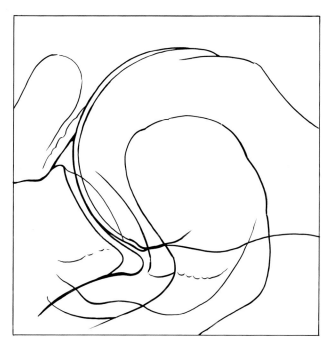

B

FIGURE 4-4. *Normal anterior glenoid labrum (small arrowheads).*

A. Trendelenburg external rotation view, which shows its inferior aspect to advantage (small white arrowhead).

B. Normal pointed anterior glenoid labrum (small black arrowhead) and rounded posterior glenoid labrum (black arrow) are both seen well on the supine axillary view, as long as excessive amounts of contrast (greater than 3 cc) are avoided.

contrast material and has a smooth concave border, which faces the humeral head (Figs. 4-1 to 4-5). The joint space is so narrow it may be completely invisible unless the patient holds a 5- or 10-pound sand bag. The upper and lower portions of the labrum are triangular and are broader than the center, giving the labrum a cup-shaped configuration (Figs. 4-1 to 4-5). The inferior surface of the superior glenoid labrum may be smooth or may have a small normal notch at its insertion with the tendon of the long head of the biceps brachii (Fig. 4-5).

The articular cartilage of the humeral head is seen on both the internal and external rotation views (Figs. 4-1A–D; 4-6). It should be uniformly smooth. There are no normal areas of flattening or irregularity along the articular surface of the humeral head.

The tendon of the long head of the biceps brachii is best seen on the standing internal and external rotation views that are obtained with soft tissue technique (Figs. 4-1C, D; 4-7). Its insertion appears as a soft tissue density originating just above the superior glenoid labrum and, as it passes through the top of the expanded capsule, it is seen as a smooth, straight soft tissue shadow (Fig. 4-7). At the level of the tuberosities, the tendon of the long head of the biceps enters an air- and contrast-filled capsular reflection referred to as the *biceps tendon sheath*. On the internal rotation view, the tendon and sheath are superimposed on the medial aspect of the humeral head. On the external rotation view, the intracapsular portions of the tendon of the long head of the biceps brachii parallels the superior aspect of the humeral head, while the intrasheath portion parallels the lateral aspect of the humeral head (Figs. 4-1A, C; 4-7A). On the external rotation view, therefore, the tendon of the long head of the biceps forms a frame along the superior and lateral aspects of the humeral head (Figs. 4-1B, D; 4-7B). On all studies, regardless of the degree of external or internal rotation, the tendon should remain in the groove created by the greater and lesser tuberosities (Figs. 4-1, 4-7).

If the synovial-lined sheath fails to fill on the pre-exercise studies, it is of little significance and adequate visualization may be achieved following exercise. If the sheath remains unfilled following exercise, it suggests that adhesions are preventing filling of the capsular reflexion, but the reason for it cannot be determined by arthrography.

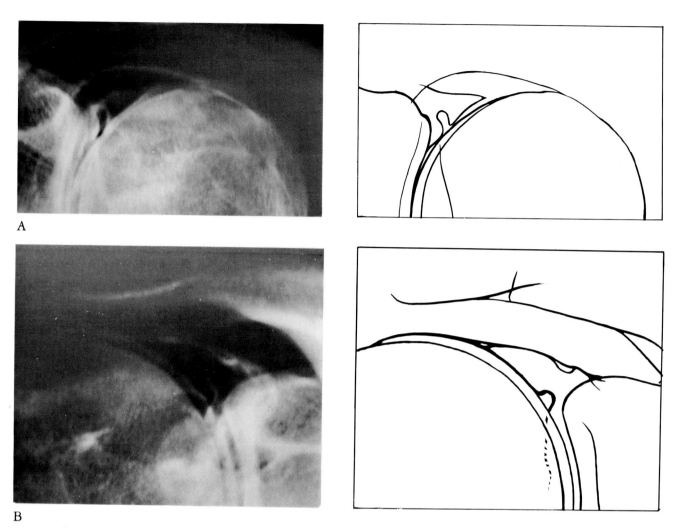

A

B

FIGURE 4-5. *Two patients (A, B) with normal notches along inferior aspect of the glenoid labrum. These indentations occur at the junction of the cartilage with the biceps tendon.*

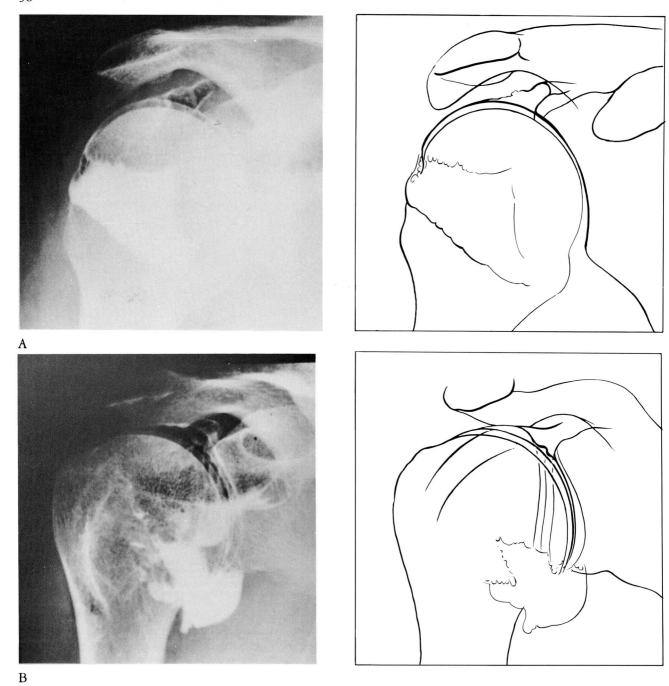

A

B

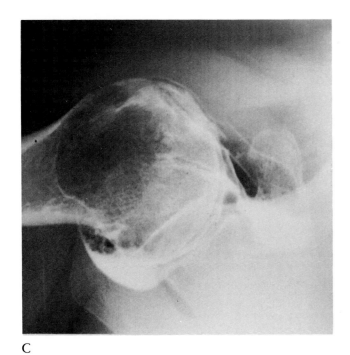

C

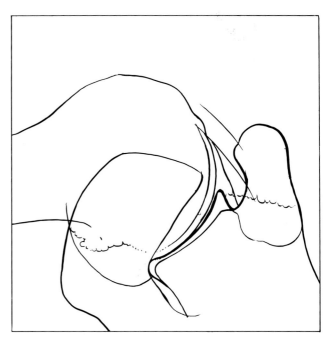

FIGURE 4-6. *Normal cartilage of humeral head.*
A thin smooth line of contrast outlines the articular
surface of the humeral head on the A, standing internal
rotation view; B, standing external rotation view; and
C, supine axillary view. There are no normal indentations in the cartilage of the humeral head.

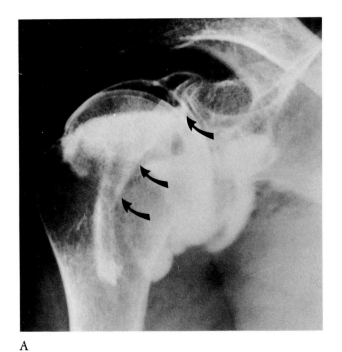

A

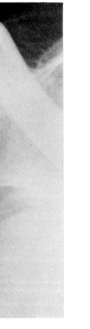

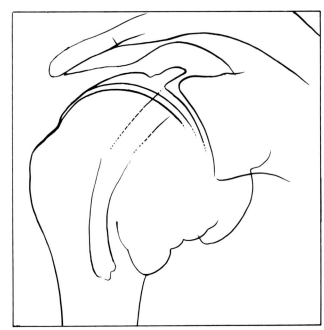

B

FIGURE 4-7. *Normal tendon of the long head of the biceps brachii (curved black arrows).*

On standing internal and external rotation views, the tendon appears as a soft tissue shadow in the air-filled capsule and contrast-filled sheath.

A. On the standing internal rotation view, the tendon is superimposed on the humeral head.

B. On the standing external rotation view, the tendon frames the superior and lateral sides of the humeral head.

Supine Axillary View

On the supine axillary view, most of the positive contrast is pooled in the posterior recess, and the pointed anterior glenoid labrum is clearly outlined by air (Figs. 4-1E, 4-3B, 4-4B). All articular surfaces of the glenoid labrum should be smooth and regular. The axillary views also demonstrate the articular cartilage of the humeral head and, as on the internal and external rotation views, it should be smooth and uniform. On the supine axillary view, the anteriorly placed bicipital groove is seen in profile, and the tendon in its sheath should be nestled between the two tuberosities (Fig. 4-1E). On the axillary view, the capsule is noted to insert along the humeral neck and no air or contrast normally crosses the proximal humeral shaft (Figs. 4-1E, 4-3B, 4-4B).

Bicipital Groove View

The tendon of the long head of the biceps is visualized en face as a round or ovoid soft tissue shadow (Fig. 4-1F). It is surrounded by the air- and contrast-filled sheath, which in turn is surrounded by the osseous groove formed by the two tuberosities. No air or contrast should be seen in the soft tissues above the bicipital groove.

Instability Series

In cases with known or suspected dislocations or subluxations of the glenohumeral joint, prone axillary [1], Stryker, and Didiee views [2] are added to the routine studies to better demonstrate the cartilaginous surfaces of the humeral head and glenoid (Fig. 4-8).

On the prone axillary view, the air rises posteriorly and outlines the posterior glenoid labrum (Fig. 4-8A). Larger than the anterior labrum, it is rounded in shape and has no sharp points or edges. The inferior glenoid labrum is also seen well on this view and is demonstrated as a smooth, unbroken line. The posterior cartilaginous articular surface of the humeral head, like its osseous surface, is smooth and rounded without any normal areas of flattening. As on the supine axillary view, no contrast crosses the proximal humeral shaft.

The Stryker view demonstrates the smooth, rounded anterior, posterior, and superior articular surfaces of the humeral head (Fig. 4-8B).

The Didiee view is another projection that further exposes the posterior surface of the humeral head and the inferior surface of the glenoid. The biceps tendon is seen extending between the tuberosities (Fig. 4-8C).

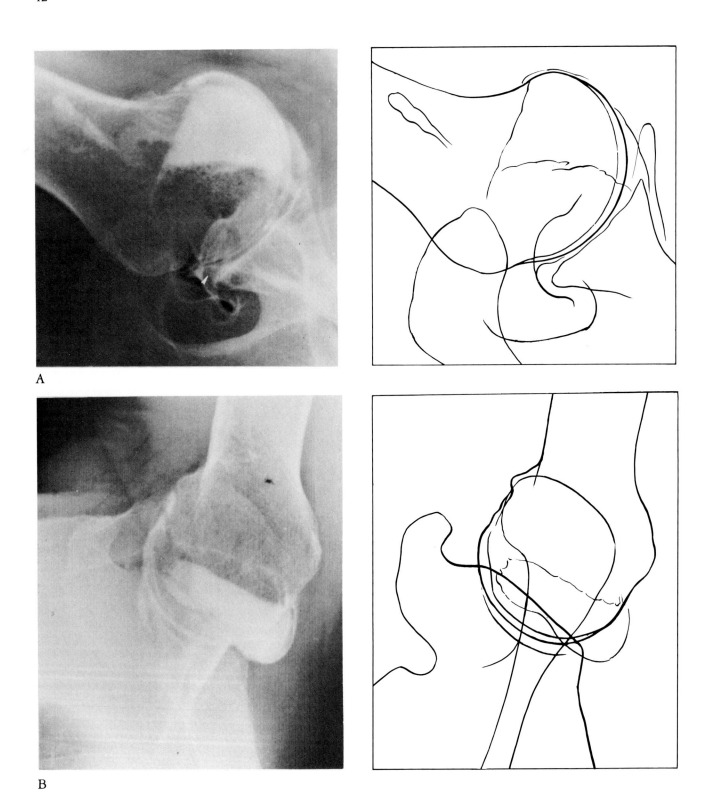

A

B

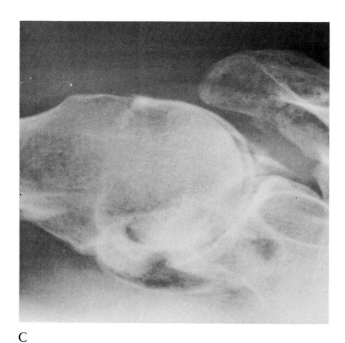

C

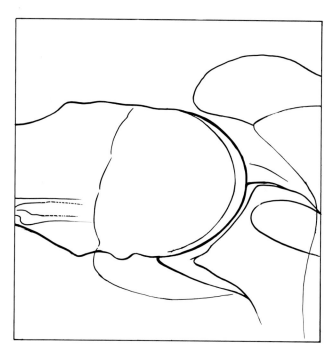

FIGURE 4-8. *Normal instability series.*

A. The prone axillary view demonstrates the rounded posterior glenoid labrum (small white arrowhead) outlined by air. The excess positive contrast pools anteriorly.

B. The notch, or Stryker view, shows the smooth uniform cartilages of the humeral head and inferior glenoid surface.

C. The Didiee view reveals the posterior articular surface of the humeral head and the inferior surface of the glenoid labrum. The biceps tendon is also seen on the projection.

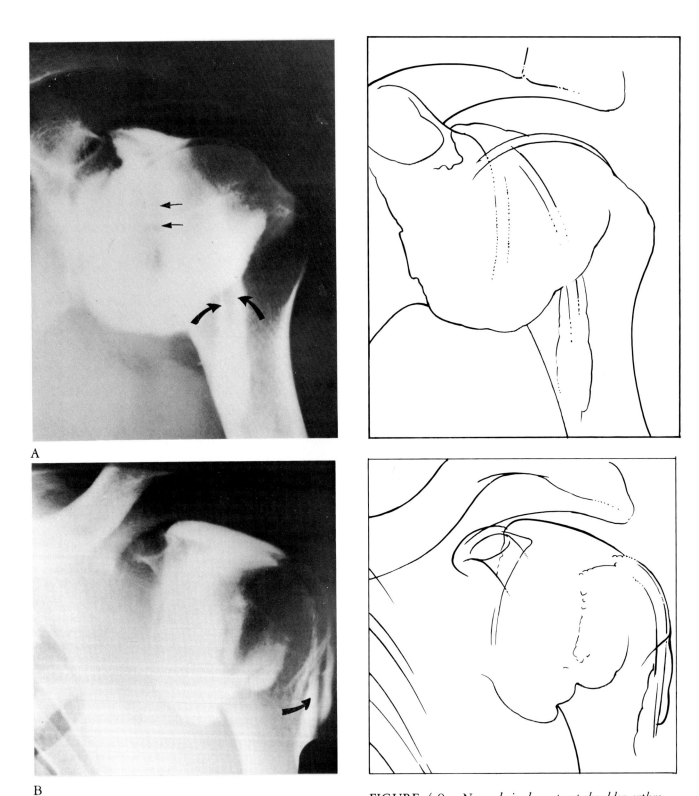

FIGURE 4-9. *Normal single contrast shoulder arthro-gram: four pre-exercise views. Supine internal and external rotation views (A, B) reveal contrast-filled capsule crossing the humeral neck.*

A. On the internal rotation view, the curvilinear radiolucency (black arrows) represents the posterior glenoid labrum seen indistinctly through the contrast. The tendon of the long head of the biceps brachii (curved black arrows) is superimposed on the humeral head and is seen as a lucency within its sheath.

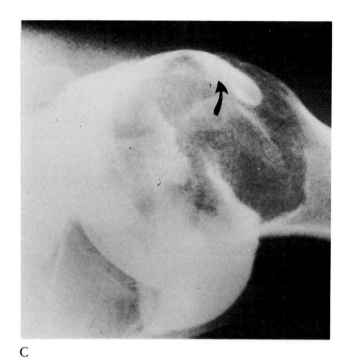

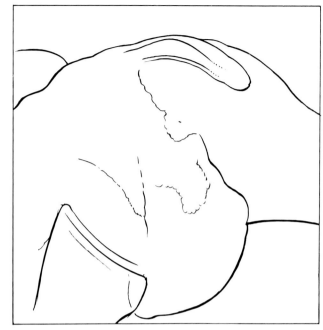

C

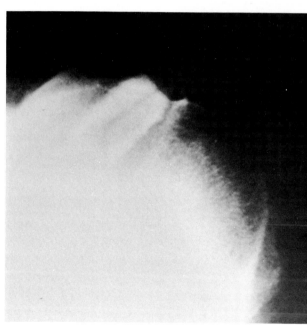

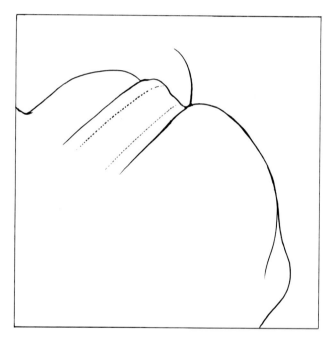

D

B. On the external rotation view, the intra-articular portion of the biceps tendon is obscured by contrast. The more distal portion of the tendon is seen within the contrast-filled sheath. Both are lateral to the humeral head (curved black arrow).

C. The supine axillary view demonstrates that no contrast crosses the proximal humeral shaft and shows the tendon of the long head of the biceps brachii in its sheath (curved black arrow). The cartilage of the glenoid is not perceptible through the contrast.

D. The bicipital groove view shows the contrast-filled biceps tendon sheath between the greater and lesser tuberosities. The margins of the lucent tendon are also obscured by the contrast material.

NORMAL SINGLE CONTRAST ARTHROGRAM

The supine internal and external rotation views obtained during a normal single contrast arthrogram demonstrate the attachment of the contrast-filled capsule to the anatomic neck of the humerus, the axillary recess hanging between the humerus and the scapula, and the subscapularis bursa resting below the coracoid process (Fig. 4-9A, B). A curvilinear radiolucency superimposed on the center of the capsule represents the posterior glenoid labrum seen indistinctly through the large amount of positive contrast material (Fig. 4-9A). On the single contrast technique, the tendon of the long head of the biceps is visualized as a radiolucency within the contrast-filled capsular reflection. Its insertion on the superior glenoid labrum and its intra-articular portion are usually poorly visualized or not visualized at all due to pooled contrast in the superior aspect of the capsule. On the internal rotation view, the tendon and sheath are superimposed on the humeral head just lateral to the shadow of the posterior glenoid labrum (Fig. 4-9A). On the external rotation view, the tendon is seen partly superimposed on the superior aspect of the humeral head, then turning inferiorly and laterally into the bicipital groove (Fig. 4-9B). A normal axillary view from a single contrast study demonstrates that no contrast crosses the proximal humeral shaft (Fig. 4-9C). A normal bicipital groove view reveals the tendon as a rounded radiolucency surrounded by positive contrast in its sheath (Fig. 4-9D). As on all four views of the double contrast study the tendon should rest between the tuberosities. The biceps tendon sheath often fails to fill with the single contrast technique. Neviaser [1] suggests that it indicates an abnormality of the tendon itself, but if the sheath fails to fill, the nature of the abnormality cannot be determined.

NORMAL EXTRAVASATION OF CONTRAST MATERIAL

With either the double or single contrast technique, the amount of contrast material injected is critical. If too much contrast medium is injected into a normal joint, there is leakage from the subscapularis bursa or axillary recess on the pre-exercise studies (Fig. 4-10A, B). These two areas are normal weak points in the joint capsule and

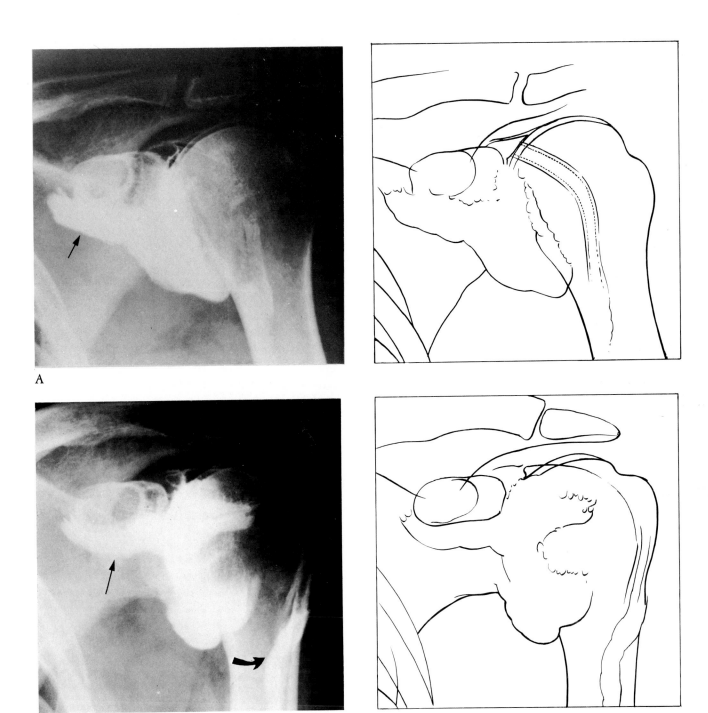

A

B

FIGURE 4-10. *Extravasation of contrast from the normal weak points in the joint capsule.*

A, B. Standing internal and external rotation views show leakage of contrast from the subscapularis bursa (black arrows) and biceps tendon sheath (curved black arrow).

extravasation should not be confused with pathology. Even when a small amount of contrast material is injected, extravasation from these sites can occur following exercise. Leakage is only significant when less than 8 cc of contrast has been injected and before any exercise. Under these conditions, an abnormally small joint capacity should be suspected.

REFERENCES

1. Neviaser, J. S. *Arthrography of the Shoulder: The Diagnosis and Management of the Lesions Visualized.* Springfield, Ill.: Thomas, 1975.
2. Rokous, J. H., Feagin, J. A., and Abbott, H. G. Modified axillary view. A useful adjunct in the diagnosis of recurrent instability of the shoulder. *Clin. Orthop.* 82:84, 1972.

SUGGESTED READING

Ghelman, B., and Goldman, A. B. The double contrast shoulder arthrogram. Evaluation of rotator cuff tears. *Radiology* 124:251, 1977.

Goldman, A. B., and Ghelman, B. The double contrast shoulder arthrogram. A review of 158 cases. *Radiology* 127:655, 1978.

Goldman, A. B. Double Contrast Shoulder Arthrography. In R. H. Freiberger and J. J. Kaye (eds.), *Arthrography.* New York: Appleton-Century-Crofts, 1979. Pp. 165–188.

Kaye, J. J., and Schneider, R. Positive Contrast Shoulder Arthrography. In R. H. Freiberger and J. J. Kaye (eds.), *Arthrography.* New York: Appleton-Century-Crofts, 1979. Pp. 109–136.

Killoran, P. J., Marcove, R. C., and Freiberger, R. H. Shoulder arthrography. *A. J. R.* 103:658, 1968.

Moseley, H. F. *Shoulder Lesions.* Baltimore: Williams & Wilkins, 1969. Pp. 37–50.

5

Tears of the Rotator Cuff

Diagnosis of a rotator cuff tear is the most common reason for ordering a shoulder arthrogram. Tightly confined between the humeral head, the acromion process, and the coracoacromial ligament, the four tendons that compose the rotator cuff are subjected to considerable mechanical stress and, therefore, varying degrees of degenerative change with loss of elasticity is the rule, rather than the exception, in patients over forty-five.

ANATOMY REVIEW

The rotator cuff is a musculotendinous hood formed by the tendons of the supraspinatus, the infraspinatus, the teres minor, and the subscapularis muscles. The first three insert on the greater tuberosity, and the subscapularis inserts on the lesser tuberosity. On its inner surface, the rotator cuff surrounds and is incorporated into the joint capsule (Fig. 5-1). Its outer surface is, in turn, covered by the subacromial-subdeltoid bursa. In a normal individual, there is no communication between the joint capsule (inside the rotator cuff) and the subacromial-subdeltoid bursa (outside the rotator cuff) (Fig. 5-1). Only a full-thickness tear of the tendons can establish such a communication.

The tendons of the cuff act together as rotators of the shoulder. In addition, they fix the humeral head in the glenoid and force it to descend in abduction. In this way, the rotator cuff maintains a fulcrum that allows the deltoid muscle to abduct the arm. The ability to abduct the arm is dependent on the depressor action of the cuff, a function that is compromised to a variable degree by tears.

PATHOPHYSIOLOGY

Rotator cuff tears can be classified into three broad categories: trauma, degeneration, and a combination of trauma and degeneration. The smallest number of cases fall into the purely traumatic group. In young individuals, a rotator cuff tear and/or detachment may follow a luxatio erecta dislocation or an anterior dislocation combined with a fracture of the greater tuberosity. However, both of these injuries are uncommon. Traumatic ruptures also occasionally result from an anterior dislocation (without significant osseous injury to the

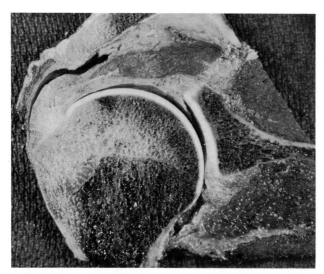

FIGURE 5-1. *Sagittal section through a gross specimen of the shoulder demonstrating the rotator cuff.*
Below the tendinous cuff is the joint capsule and joint space. Above the rotator cuff is the narrow space formed by the subacromial-subdeltoid bursa. The insertion of the rotator cuff is identified at the tuberosities.

humeral head) or following a severe soft tissue contusion.

The second group of rotator cuff tears consists of degenerative lesions in elderly individuals. Frequently seen as incidental findings on chest roentgenograms, they are not associated with a specific traumatic incident.

The third and largest category of rotator cuff tears is attributable to the combination of trauma and degenerative changes that occurs in middle-aged individuals. A tear may result from a gradual wearing through of the tendons or may occur following a fall or after lifting a heavy object. Regardless of the type of insult, the superimposed trauma produces a rent in the already compromised tendons.

Tears of the rotator cuff vary in severity from minor interruptions of a few fibers to massive disruptions of the whole cuff. The most common site of injury or "critical zone" is at the insertion of the supraspinatus tendon on the greater tuberosity [1]. It has been suggested that after the fifth decade of life, compromise of the blood supply to this area renders the tendons particularly susceptible to attritional changes.

When the rotator cuff is damaged, the humeral head impinges on the coracoacromial arch producing pain, decreased range of motion, and decreased power. The deltoid loses its biomechanical advantage, exacerbating the loss of mobility and strength [4]. With large tears, the cuff loses its depressor action and no longer acts as a fulcrum about which the deltoid can elevate the arm.

An injury to the rotator cuff triggers a self-perpetuating cycle of damage referred to as the *impingement syndrome.* Originally called the "supraspinatus syndrome" by Codman [1], and the "painful arc" by Watson-Jones [2], this entity was extensively researched and renamed by Neer [4]. The impingement syndrome encompasses a spectrum of abnormalities that result in faulty excursion of the humeral head under the coracoacromial arch. Both a rotator cuff tear and abnormality of the tendon of the long head of the biceps brachii can lead to alterations in joint mechanics and an imbalance in muscle pull. The unopposed deltoid then forces the humeral head upward, and when the arm is held in variable degrees of abduction, the tuberosities impinge on the coracoacromial arch and create pain (Fig. 5-2). Further abduction can only be achieved through scapular motion and

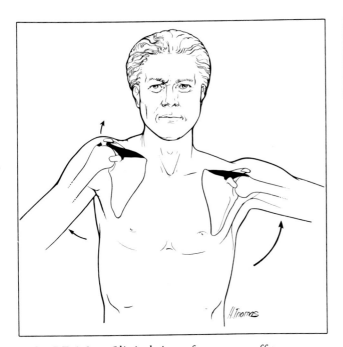

FIGURE 5-2.   *Clinical signs of a rotator cuff tear.*
Patients with rotator cuff tears abduct the arm via scapular motion and a shrugging movement. Pain and weakness are most evident when abducting the arm against passive resistance. The humeral head has moved upward due to the unopposed force of the deltoid.

a shrugging movement. The rotator cuff and the tendon of the long head of the biceps are then exposed to repetitive trauma, producing edema, inflammation, and further degeneration. This, in turn, leads to thickening of the ligaments and further limitation of the range of motion of the humeral head. The end result of this vicious cycle are osseous changes in the undersurface of the acromion, adhesive capsulitis secondary to adhesions, and lastly, complete attrition of the tendinous structures.

CLINICAL

Rotator cuff tears occur most frequently in the sixth decade of life and are more common in males than in females. There is a higher incidence of this injury in individuals whose work requires heavy lifting or climbing. The course of the pain is variable, and it may begin as minimal discomfort and gradually progress to higher intensity. Limitation of motion may be gradual, or may occur suddenly following a direct blow to the shoulder or from lifting a heavy object. In young persons, the onset is almost always acute following a significant injury to the shoulder.

The physical examination demonstrates pain on active motion, limitation of active and/or passive motion, and tenderness above the humeral head or tuberosities. Pain and weakness is most evident in abduction against active resistance, and the "drop arm test" is positive (Fig. 5-2). This test is performed by passively abducting the affected arm above the horizontal and releasing it to determine whether the patient is able to maintain the abduction without support. Inability to perform the test is suggestive of a rotator cuff tear, but not conclusive, as referred pain may produce a similar result. The accuracy of the drop arm test is increased if it follows the injection of local anesthesia into the area of maximal tenderness. Approximately 3 weeks after an injury, atrophy of the supraspinatus or infraspinatus may also be evident at physical examination.

Unfortunately, because of the close anatomic relationship between the rotator cuff and the surrounding structures, a specific diagnosis is difficult to establish on the basis of a physical examination. The clinical differential diagnosis includes calcific peritendinitis, subacromial bursitis, acute abnormalities of the tendon of the long head of the biceps brachii, and degenerative changes in the acromioclavicular joint.

Both single and double contrast arthrograms provide an accurate means of demonstrating rotator cuff tears. The double contrast technique also demonstrates the presence of preexisting degenerative changes in the tendons and helps distinguish between acute and chronic tears.

PLAIN FILMS

For most patients with rotator cuff tears, the plain films are negative or nonspecific. If, however, the changes are chronic and long-standing, routine views can demonstrate the following (Fig. 5-3):

1. A decrease in the distance between the humeral head and the acromion process
2. "Faceting" of the undersurface of the acromion (sclerosis and loss of its normal convex undersurface)
3. Cystic changes, and/or sclerosis adjacent to the tuberosities

At the Hospital for Special Surgery, experience has shown that positive plain film findings occur late in the course of the disease, and the subsequent arthrogram usually reveals either complete absence of the rotator cuff or only a few small detached remnants.

ARTHROGRAPHIC ABNORMALITIES DIAGNOSTIC OF ROTATOR CUFF TEARS

The term *complete rotator cuff tear* does not refer to rupture of all four tendons. Rather, it indicates an interruption that extends through the entire width of one or more of the four muscles (Fig. 5-4). A complete tear of the rotator cuff establishes an abnormal connection between the joint capsule on its inner surface and the subacromial-subdeltoid bursa on its superior surface. The term *partial rotator cuff tear* refers to an interruption that does not extend through the full width of the cuff (Fig. 5-4A, B, C). Partial tears can occur either in the superior or inferior surfaces of the cuff or in the substance of the tendons. However, the only partial tears that can be diagnosed by shoulder arthrography are those that involve the inferior surface of the rotator cuff and therefore tear the capsule as well.

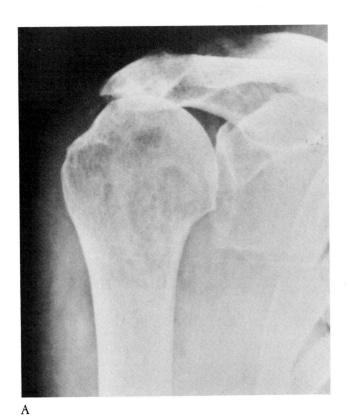

A

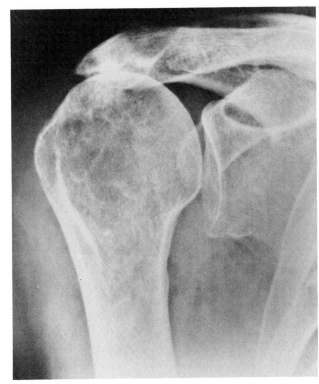

B

FIGURE 5-3.   *Plain film criteria of a chronic rotator cuff tear.*

A, B. Internal and external rotation views show less than an 8-millimeter distance between the humeral head and acromion process. There is "faceting" or an abnormal concavity of the undersurface of the acromion. Cystic lucencies are present at the base of the tuberosities.

54

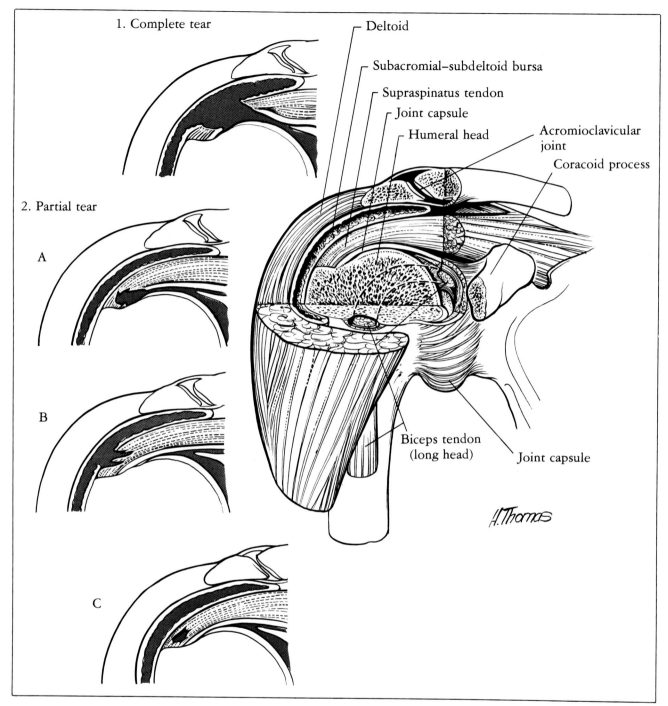

1. Complete tear

Deltoid

Subacromial–subdeltoid bursa

Supraspinatus tendon

Joint capsule

Humeral head

Acromioclavicular joint

Coracoid process

2. Partial tear

A

B

Biceps tendon (long head)

Joint capsule

C

H. Thomas

FIGURE 5-4. *Types of rotator cuff tears.*
A complete rotator cuff tear, by definition, extends through the full vertical width of the cuff and establishes an abnormal communication between the joint capsule below and the subacromial-subdeltoid bursa above. Partial tears do not extend through the full vertical width of the cuff. They may occur on the inferior surface of the tendons, A, in the body of the tendons, B, or on the superior surface of the tendons, C. Only the partial tears on the inferior surface of the cuff will tear the capsule, A, and be diagnosed on shoulder arthrography.

The single arthrographic criterion of a complete rotator cuff tear is visualization of injected contrast material extending from the capsule into the subacromial-subdeltoid bursa. On the internal and external rotation views, contrast material is seen below the acromion process (subacromial bursa), lateral to the articular cartilage of the humeral head, and below the greater tuberosity (subdeltoid bursa). Contrast material in any or all of these locations indicates a complete rupture of the rotator cuff (Figs. 5-5 to 5-19). In some patients, adhesions can confine the contrast material to one site, but the diagnosis can still be established as long as the contrast is seen in one of these abnormal locations (Fig. 5-10). Extension of contrast from the subacromial bursa into the acromioclavicular joint, the *geiser sign* [4, 5], suggests that the tear is long-standing (Fig. 5-8A). On the axillary view, a collection of contrast is seen crossing the proximal humeral shaft (subdeltoid bursa) (Fig. 5-8B), and on the bicipital groove view, air or contrast or both are noted above the tendon and tuberosities (subdeltoid bursa) (Fig. 5-13). If an abnormality of the tendon of the long head of the biceps coexists with the rotator cuff tear, an "impingement syndrome" can be suspected (Fig. 5-13).

Partial rotator cuff tears are identified arthrographically when abnormal collections of contrast extend above the articular cartilage of the humeral head or above the line of the joint capsule, but do not reach the acromion process superiorly or the tuberosities inferiorly (Figs. 5-20 to 5-22). The optimum projection for the diagnosis of partial rotator cuff tears is the internal rotation view. On the external rotation projection, the superimposed tendon of the long head of the biceps may obscure small partial tears. The axillary and bicipital groove views are negative with a partial tear.

Accurate diagnosis of both partial and complete tears of the rotator cuff depend largely on the performance of postexercise studies (Fig. 5-22B). Without postexercise studies, tears may be entirely missed or incomplete tears may be mistakenly diagnosed as partial tears.

Once the diagnosis of a rotator cuff tear has been established, two decisions in clinical management remain: first, the choice of surgical candidates and second, in operative cases, the choice of the best surgical incision to achieve a tension-free repair.

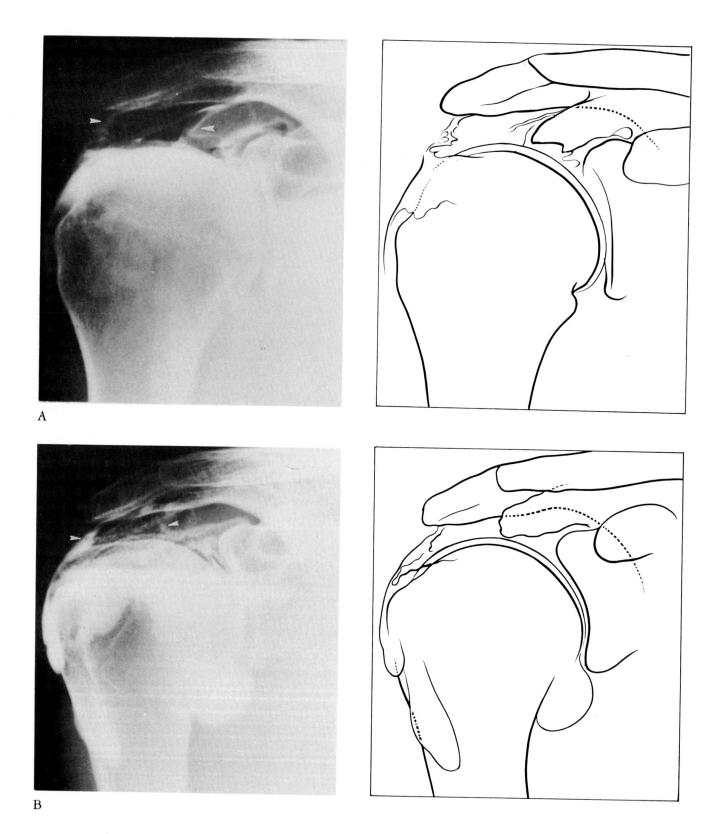

A

B

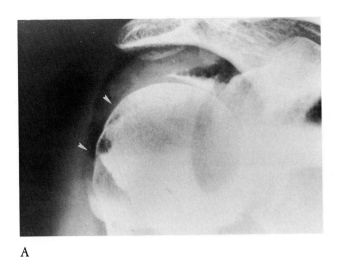

A

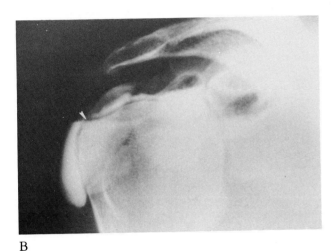

B

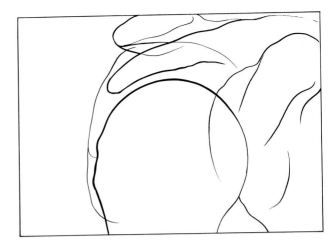

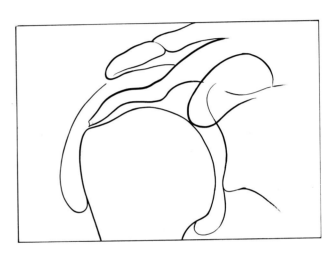

◀ FIGURE 5-5. *Complete rotator cuff tear.*

A, B. Standing internal and external rotation views show contrast extending from the capsule to the space just below the acromion process (subacromial bursa). On the internal rotation view, A, positive contrast is noted lateral to the humeral head and below the tuberosities (subdeltoid bursa). On both projections the tear is noted to be wide (white arrowheads), and the fragments of the cuff are smooth and of normal width.

Sources: Goldman, A. B. and Ghelman, B. The double contrast shoulder arthrogram. A review of 158 cases. *Radiology* 127:655, 1978. With permission; Goldman, A. B. Double Contrast Shoulder Arthrography. In R. H. Freiberger and J. J. Kaye (Eds.), *Arthrography.* New York: Appleton-Century-Crofts, 1979.

FIGURE 5-6. *Complete rotator cuff tear.*

A, B. Standing internal and external rotation views reveal air and contrast beneath the acromion process, and below the tuberosities. The tear is moderate in width (white arrowheads). The fragments of the tendinous cuff are smooth and occupy most of the space between the cartilage of the humeral head and the acromion process.

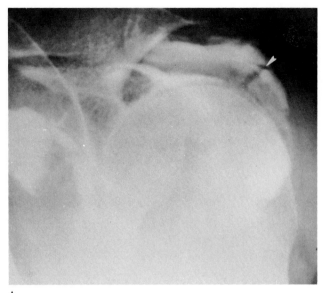
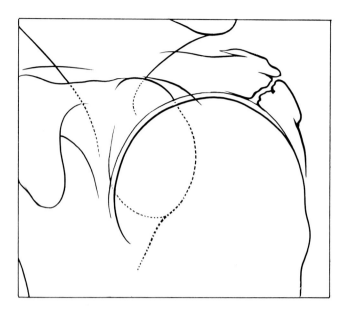

A

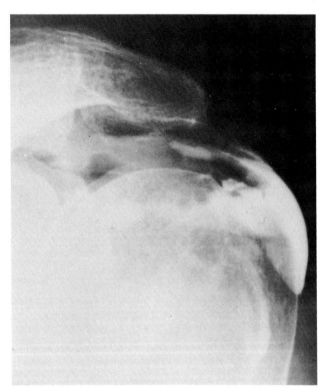
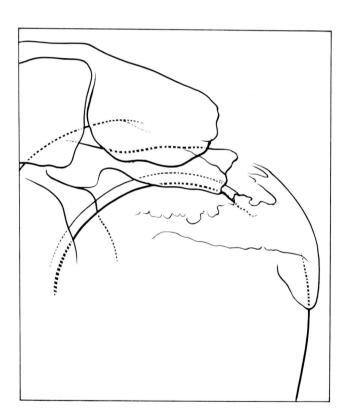

B

FIGURE 5-7. *Complete rotator cuff tear.*

A, B. Standing internal and external rotation views demonstrating a narrow tear (white arrowhead). The tendinous cuff is still of normal width occupying the space between the cartilage of the humeral head and the acromion process.

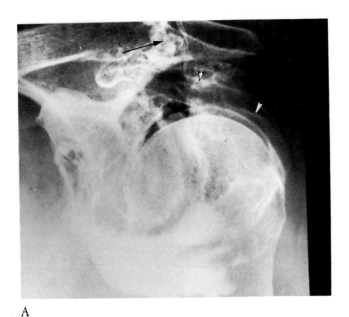

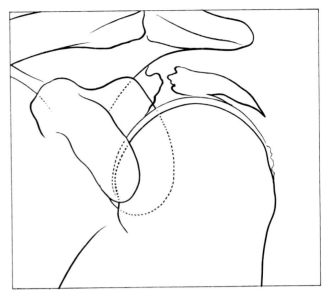

A

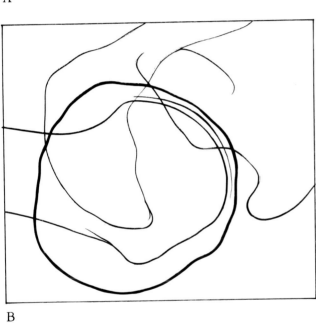

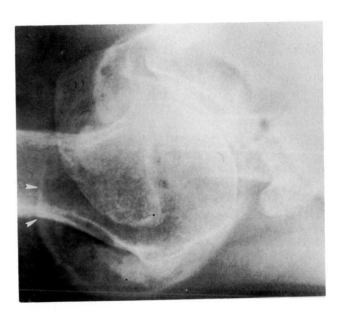

B

FIGURE 5-8.   *Complete rotator cuff tear.*

A. The standing internal rotation view shows a complex complete rotator cuff tear with at least two lines of contrast extending through the substance of the tendons (white arrowheads). Note contrast also extending into the acromioclavicular joint (black arrow).

B. The axillary view reveals an abnormal collection of contrast crossing the proximal humeral shaft (subdeltoid bursa) (white arrowheads).

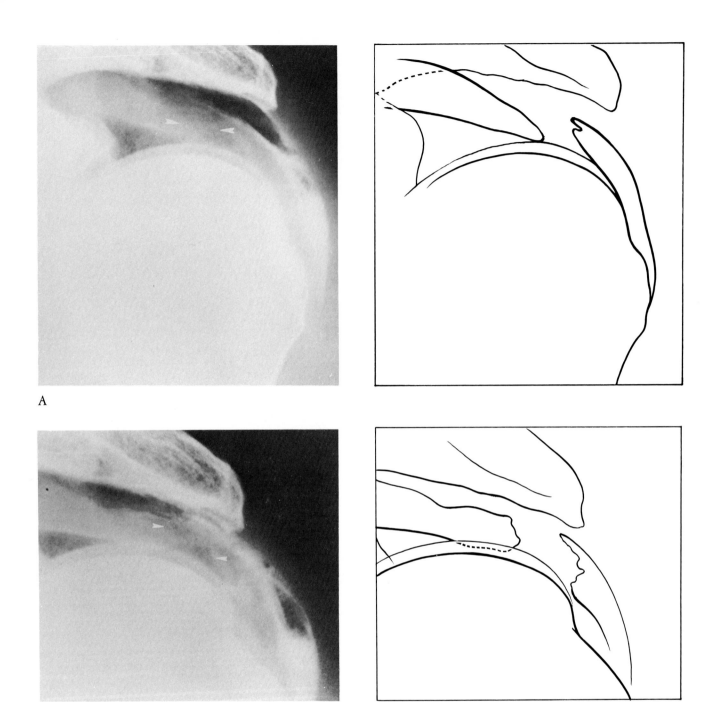

A

B

FIGURE 5-9. *Complete rotator cuff tear.*

A, B. Standing internal and external rotation views demonstrate a complete but narrow tear (white arrowheads). Since some tissue remains behind or in front of the tear, it does not appear completely lucent.

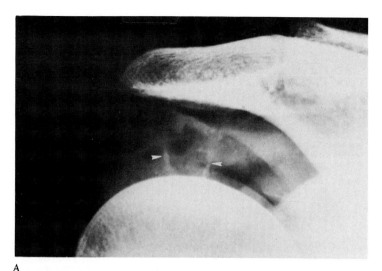
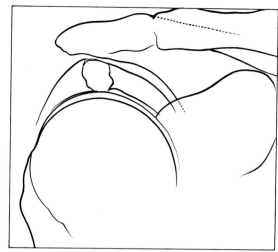

A

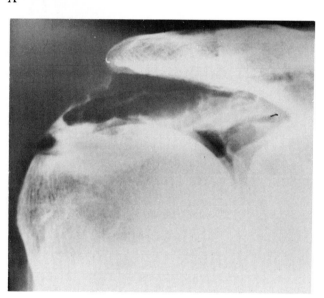
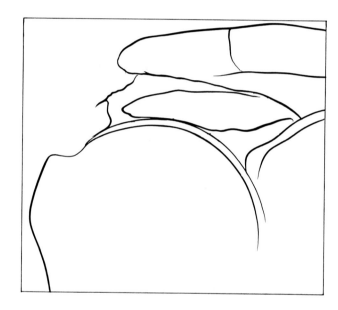

B

FIGURE 5-10.   *Complete rotator cuff tear.*

A, B. Standing internal and external rotation views
show air extending from the capsule, through a
complete rotator cuff tear (white arrowheads),
and into the space below the acromion process
(subacromial bursa). The superior surface of the
rotator cuff can only be seen if a tear is present.
The width of the tendinous fragments are normal. In this case no contrast extends into the
subdeltoid bursa, either because of adhesions or
edema.

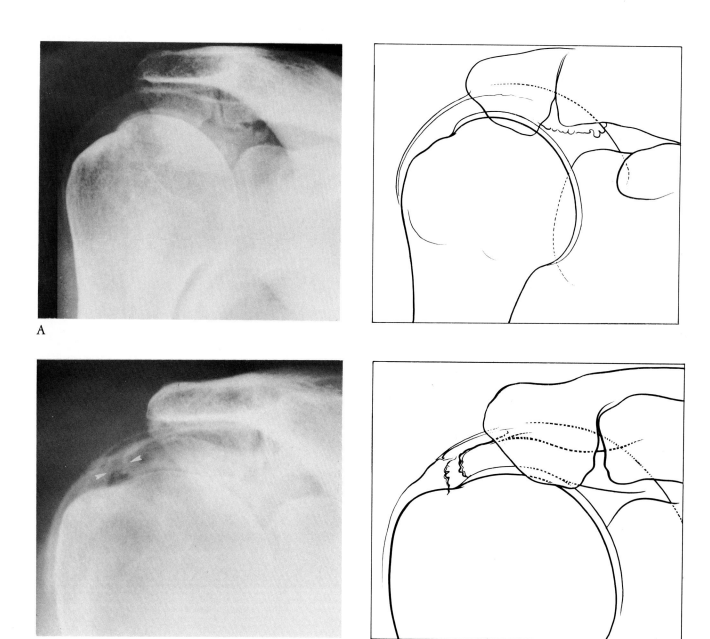

A

B

FIGURE 5-11. *Complete rotator cuff tear.*

A, B. Standing internal and external rotation views demonstrate abnormal collections of contrast below the acromion process, lateral to the humeral head, and below the tuberosities. In this case the tear itself (white arrowheads) is seen only on the external rotation view, B.

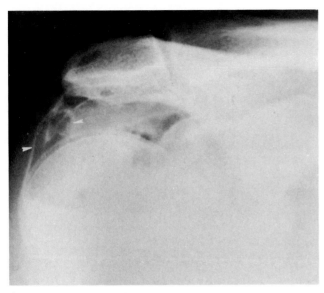

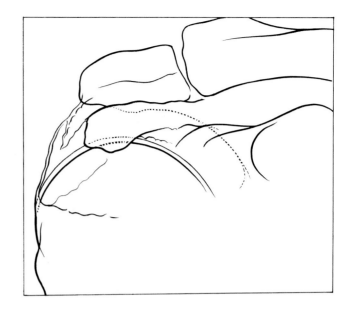

A

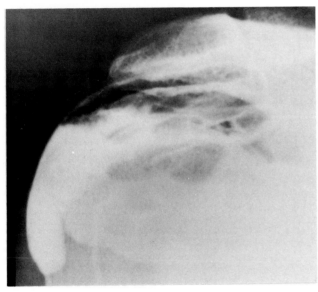

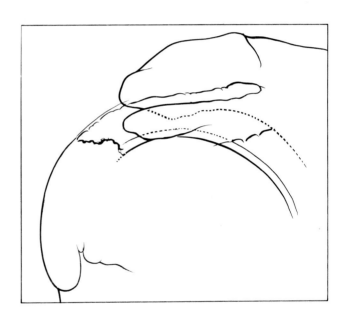

B

FIGURE 5-12.   *Complete rotator cuff tear.*

A, B. Standing internal and external rotation views
demonstrate a narrow tear (white arrowheads)
that occurred at the insertion of the supraspinatus tendon on the greater tuberosity. Owing to its poor vascular supply, this site is particularly at risk and is referred to as the "critical
area." The tendinous fragments are of normal
width and occupy the space between the cartilage of the humeral head and the acromion process.

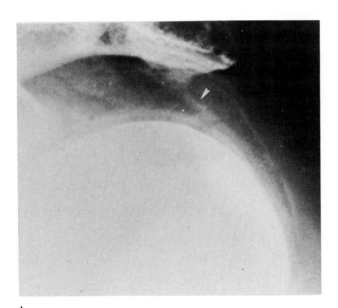

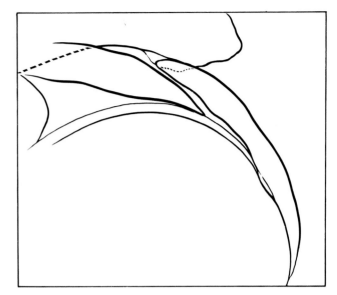

A

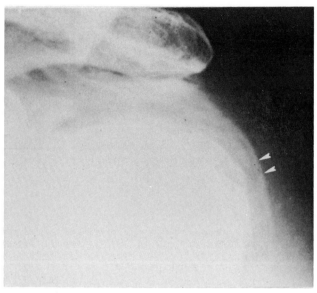

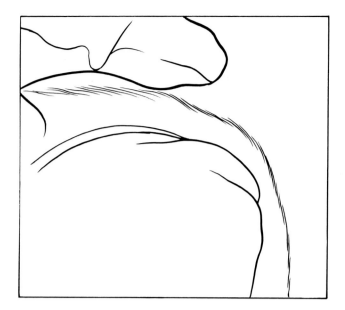

B

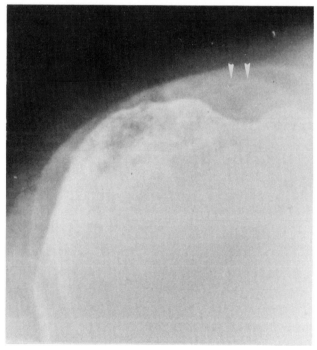

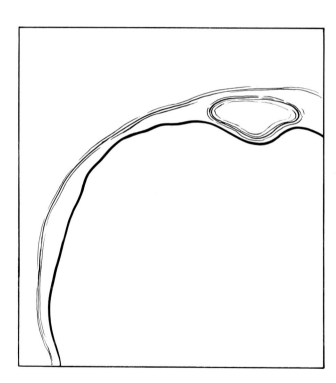

C

FIGURE 5-13. *Impingement syndrome.*

A. The standing internal rotation view shows a narrow oblique complete rotator cuff tear (white arrowhead). Contrast is within the subacromial-subdeltoid bursa.

B, C. The standing external rotation view and bicipital groove view demonstrates swelling of the tendon of the long head of the biceps brachii (double white arrowheads). The tendon occupies the entire sheath and the margins of the sheath are poorly defined (double white arrowheads).

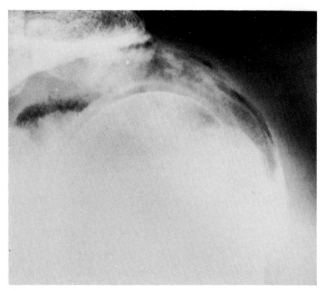

A

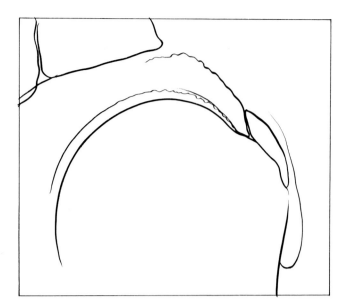

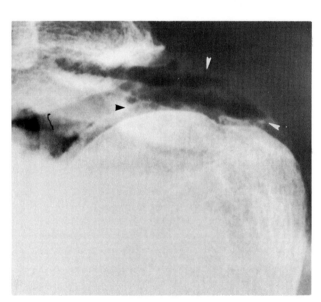

B

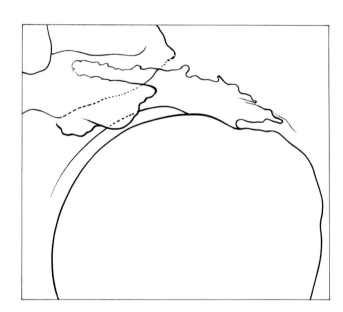

FIGURE 5-14. *Complete rotator cuff tear with degenerative changes in tendons.*

A, B. Standing internal and external rotation views show contrast below the acromion process (subacromial bursa) lateral to the humeral head and below the tuberosities (subdeltoid bursa). The remaining cuff still occupies most of the space between the cartilage of the humeral head and acromion process, but the margins of the tendons (arrowheads) are ragged and irregular.

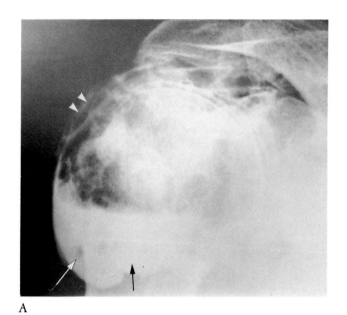

A

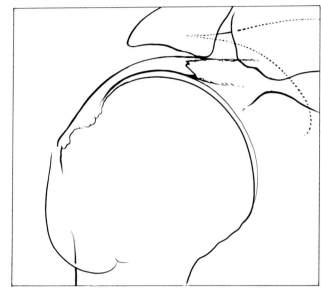

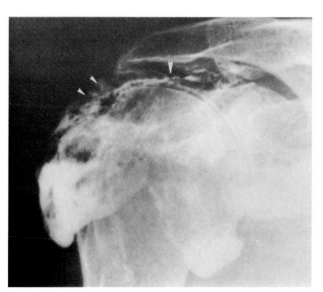

B

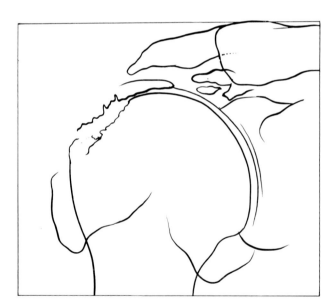

FIGURE 5-15. *Complete rotator cuff tear with degenerative changes in the tendons.*

A, B. Standing internal and external rotation views reveal multiple tears (white arrowheads) and irregularity of the surfaces of the torn tendons. The soft tissue shadow of the cuff no longer occupies the entire space between the cartilage of the humeral head and the acromion process. The subacromial-subdeltoid bursa is expanded suggesting chronicity (arrows).

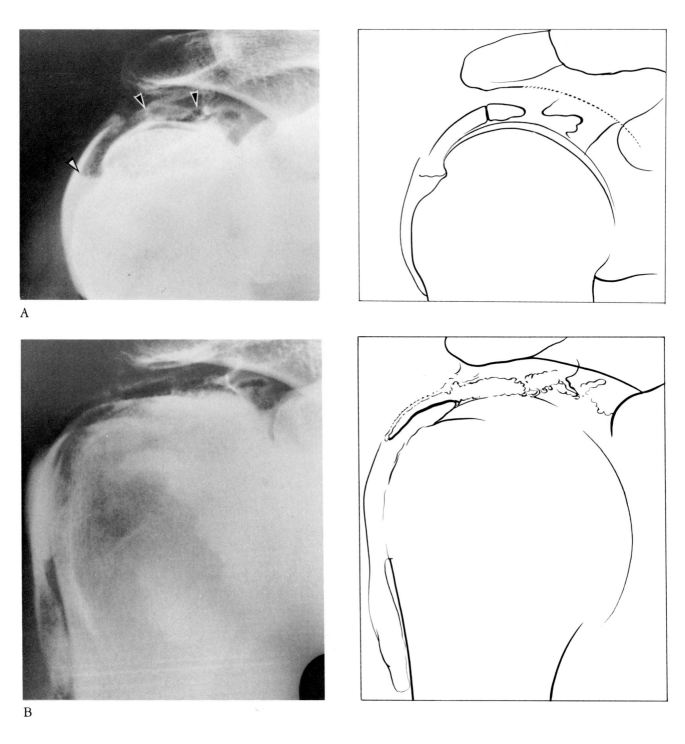

A

B

FIGURE 5-16. *Complete rotator cuff tear with degenerative changes in the tendons.*

A, B. Standing internal and external rotation views show several lines of contrast extending through the soft tissue shadow of the rotator cuff (arrowheads). Both the superior and inferior sides of the tendinous cuff are outlined by contrast because of the complete tears. The remaining cuff is narrow and irregular.

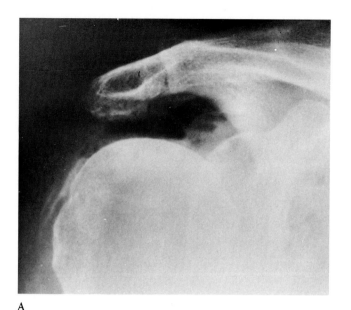

A

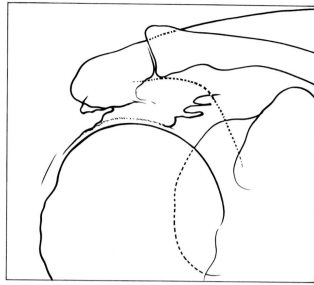

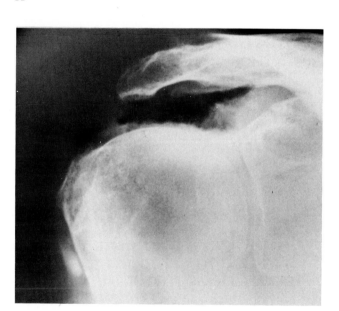

B

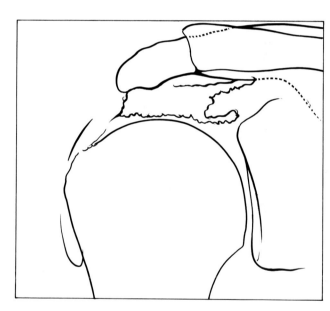

FIGURE 5-17.   *Complete rotator cuff tear with degenerative changes in the tendons.*

A, B. Standing internal and external rotation views show an extremely wide rotator cuff tear with half of the superior articular surface of the humeral head uncovered. The ends of the tendons are frayed.

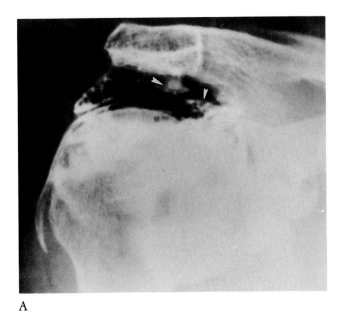

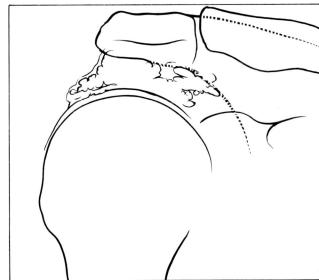

A

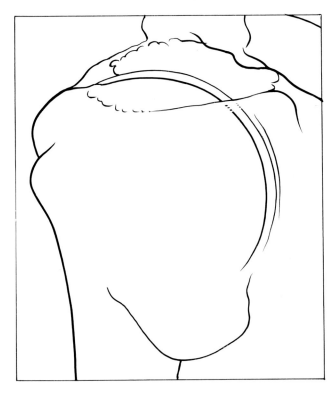

B

FIGURE 5-18. *Complete rotator cuff tear with degenerative changes in the tendons.*

A, B. Standing internal and external rotation views reveal only small soft tissue fragments (white arrowheads) between the cartilage of the humeral head and the acromion process. The superior articular surface of the humerus is denuded.

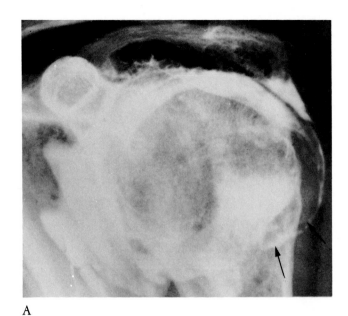

A

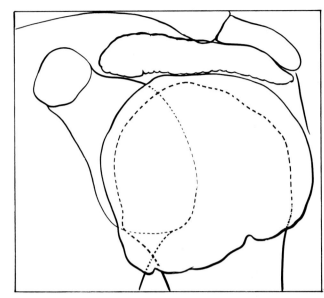

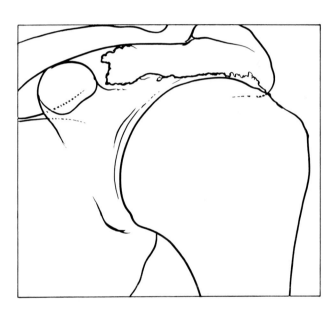

B

FIGURE 5-19.   *Complete rotator cuff tear with degeneration of the tendons.*

A, B.   Standing internal and external rotation views show only air and contrast above the humeral head. No soft tissue tendon cuff is visualized. The subacromial-subdeltoid bursa is enlarged and patulous (black arrows) due to the chronicity of the rotator cuff tear.

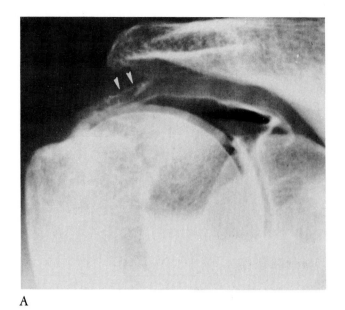

A

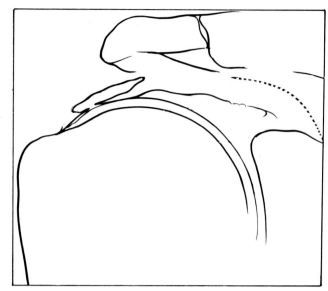

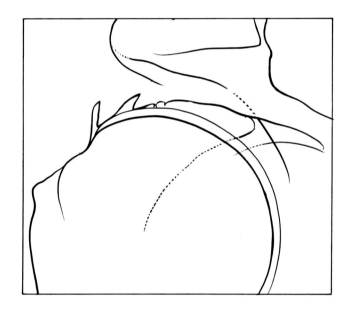

B

FIGURE 5-20. *Partial rotator cuff tear.*

A, B. Standing internal and external rotation views reveal an abnormal collection of contrast extending above the cartilage of the humeral head (white arrowheads) but not all the way to the acromion process.

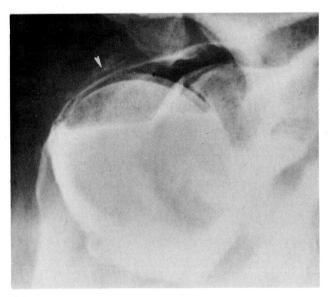

A

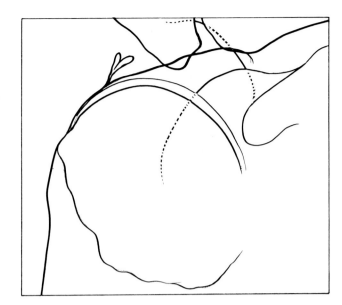

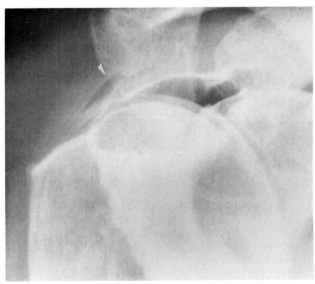

B

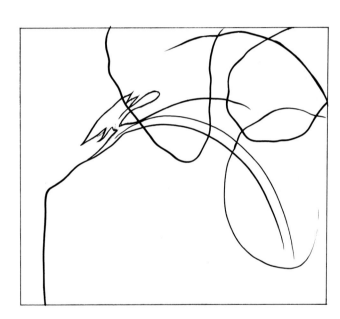

FIGURE 5-21. *Partial rotator cuff tear.*

A. A pre-exercise internal rotation view shows a small abnormal collection of contrast above the cartilage of the humeral head (white arrowhead).

B. A postexercise study demonstrates an enlargement of the abnormal shadow (white arrowhead), but it remains confined to the inferior portion of the cuff and no contrast reaches the subacromial bursa or the top of the rotator cuff.

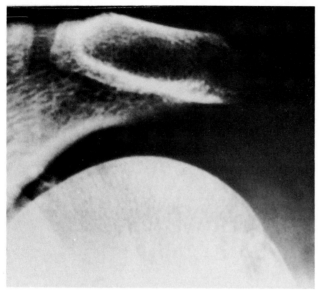
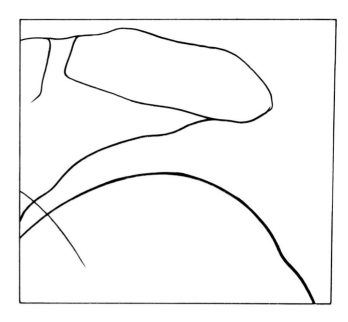

A

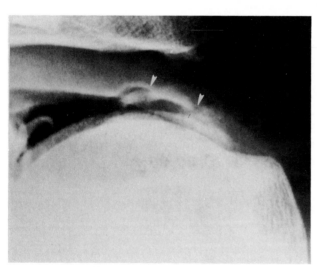
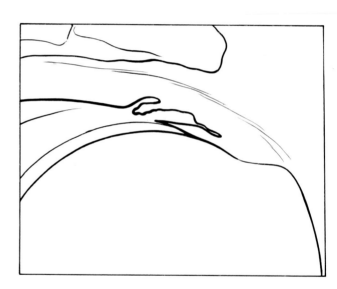

B

FIGURE 5-22. *Partial rotator cuff tear.*

A. A pre-exercise standing internal rotation view demonstrates poor coating of the top of the capsule.

B. A postexercise standing internal rotation view demonstrates better coating and a large partial tear of the inferior surface of the rotator cuff (white arrowheads).

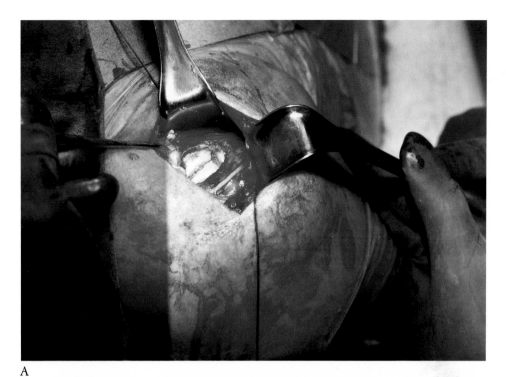

A

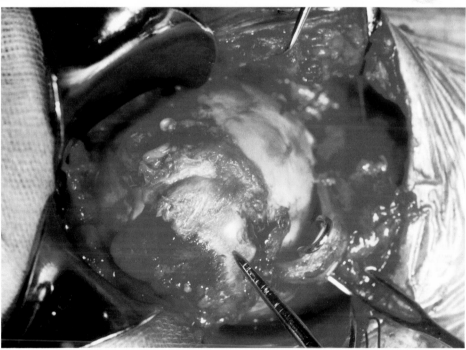

B

FIGURE 5-23. *Surgical examples of complete rotator cuff tears.*

A. Complete tear seen extending into the superior surface of the cuff. The surrounding tendons are of good quality.

B. Complete tear with associated degenerative changes in the tendons.

Indications for surgery include acute traumatic tears (Fig. 5-23A) or chronic tears that have been treated with a course of conservative therapy but still produce pain and weakness. The principal contraindication for a primary repair of the rotator cuff is severe degeneration of the tendons that leaves, as McLaughlin [3] describes it, "only rotten cloth to sew" (Fig. 5-23B). The double contrast technique has the advantage over the single contrast technique of coating the fragments of the torn cuff and demonstrating both the quality of the remaining tissues and the width of the tear itself. These tears are best evaluated on standing internal and external rotation views obtained with the soft tissue technique (Figs. 5-5 to 5-19). The arthrographic criteria for degenerative changes illustrated in Figures 5-4 to 5-19 are as follows:

1. Irregularity of the surfaces of the torn tendons
2. Narrowing of the disrupted tendons (a normal rotator cuff should occupy the majority of the space between the articular cartilage of the humeral head and the osseous acromion process)
3. Air or contrast within the fragments themselves (an indication of multiple rents as opposed to a single tear)
4. Complete absence of the soft tissue shadow of the rotator cuff.

Tears of the rotator cuff associated with rheumatoid arthritis have a somewhat different arthrographic appearance. In these patients, the tendinous cuff has an irregular inferior surface and appears to be diffusely narrowed beginning from its glenohumeral side. A full-width tear may or may not be present, depending on the duration of the arthritis in the glenohumeral joint and on whether the acromioclavicular joint is also affected.

Visualization of the fragments of the rotator cuff also permits evaluation of the width of the tear. If the donut is visualized, so is the hole (Figs. 5-5 to 5-19). The width of the tear is reported as the percent of the humeral head that is not covered by the rotator cuff. Knowing the width of the tear can be important in identifying cases with severe retraction, which would make a primary repair technically difficult.

Following a successful repair of the rotator cuff, the arthrogram should be essentially normal. There may be some irregularities in the contour of the joint capsule, but the contrast should not be seen outside of the confines of the capsule.

CAUSES OF MISINTERPRETATION

Most false-positive studies result from the interpretation of normal structures as abnormal tears. On the external rotation view, the tendon of the long head of the biceps and its air- and contrast-filled sheath are superimposed on the inferior portion of the rotator cuff and may be mistaken for a tear (Fig. 5-24A). The course of the tendon, framing the superior and lateral aspects of the humeral head, and its smooth linear contour should differentiate it from contrast within the substance of the rotator cuff. However, even more definitive is the observation that the internal rotation and axillary views are negative.

A second normal structure, which may be misinterpreted as a rotator cuff tear, is the capsular recess between the medial insertion of the capsule and the superior glenoid labrum (Fig. 5-24B). The capsule normally inserts proximal to the fibrous rim of the glenoid so that air and/or contrast should be seen extending above the superior aspect of the fibrous and cartilage rim. This collection can be differentiated from a partial tear of the rotator cuff because of its medial location on both the internal and external rotation views (the vast majority of partial tears are lateral and occur adjacent to the greater tuberosity), its triangular shape, and its smooth superior surface, which is continuous with the outline of the capsule.

A third normal structure is the fat line, which frequently outlines the superior surface of the rotator cuff on the internal and external rotation views (Fig. 5-24C). This normal structure is best seen on films obtained with soft-tissue technique. In some individuals this lucency may be prominent and may be mistaken for air in the subacromial bursa. Absence of positive contrast leakage, absence of air in the subdeltoid bursa, and the presence of this lucency on the plain films differentiate the normal fat pad from an abnormal rotator cuff tear.

False-positive studies can also result from the misinterpretation of plain film findings as abnormalities of the contrast study. Calcium in the supraspinatus tendon can occasionally mimic contrast in the rotator cuff (Fig. 5-25A). A lipoma may rarely be mistaken for air outside of the capsule (Fig. 5-25B). Comparison with a preliminary film should eliminate this type of error.

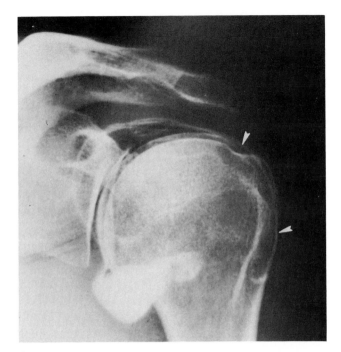

A

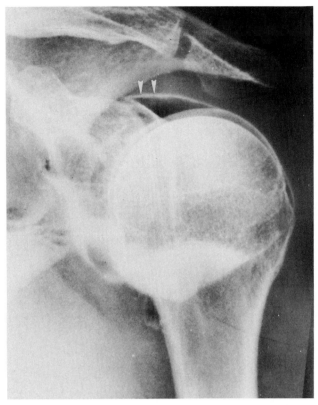

B

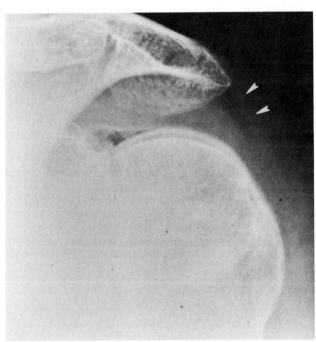

C

FIGURE 5-24. *Normal structures that can be mistaken for rotator cuff tears.*

A. The tendon of the long head of the biceps brachii, on the external rotation view, produces a shadow above and lateral to the humeral head (white arrowheads). On the internal rotation view, B, the tendon is rotated medially and away from the area of the rotator cuff.

B. The normal recess above the superior glenoid labrum (white arrowheads) is seen on both internal and external rotation views. Its medial position, above the glenoid, should distinguish it from abnormal rotator cuff tears, which occur more laterally and over the humeral head.

C. A normal fat pad (white arrowheads) can be seen outlining the superior surface of the rotator cuff. It is not as lucent as air and, of course, there is no positive contrast in the area.

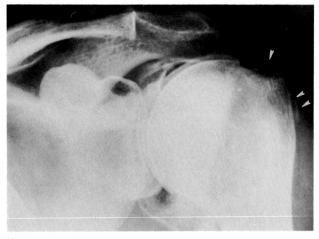

A

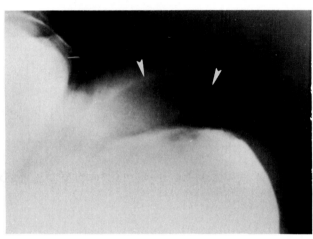

B

FIGURE 5-25. *Plain film abnormalities that mimic a rotator cuff tear.*
These include, A, calcific tendinitis (white arrowheads) and, B, a lipoma (white arrowheads). Comparison with scout films should eliminate confusion.

The most unusual cause for a false-positive shoulder arthrogram is the inadvertent injection of contrast material into the subacromial or subdeltoid bursa (Fig. 5-26). In normal individuals this structure is a potential space. However, if there is surrounding inflammation or bursitis, the space may become sufficiently dilated so that if filled with contrast, it can mimic the joint capsule. On the internal and external rotation views, contrast is seen superimposed on the glenohumeral joint and also extending up to the acromion process. However, the axillary view clearly demonstrates that there is no contrast within the joint space itself.

Most false-negative shoulder arthrograms result from a failure to perform adequate postexercise studies. Another less common reason is severe coexisting adhesive capsulitis. In the most severe cases of frozen shoulder, all of the contrast material extravasates through the subscapularis bursa before films can be obtained (Fig. 5-27). In such instances, no conclusion as to the status of the rotator cuff can be drawn.

The last problem in interpretation occurs specifically with the double contrast technique. In 2 of 381 cases reported by the authors, a small amount of air was observed beneath the acromion process. Despite multiple postexercise studies, no positive contrast entered the subacromial-subdeltoid bursa, the amount of extravasated air did not increase, and the interruption in the cuff itself was never visualized. In one instance, surgery revealed a small tear of approximately one-half centimeter in diameter. In the second, no obvious tear was identified at exploration. This minimal leakage of air into the subacromial bursa probably reflects a small interruption in the cuff, which may or may not be of clinical significance. A follow-up study after a period of conservative treatment is advised.

TREATMENT

Treatment of rotator cuff tears depends on several factors, including the age of the patient, the duration of symptoms, and the functional impairment. The size of the tear also influences the treatment plan. At one end of the spectrum are young to middle-aged patients with a history of recent trauma who sustain acute tears. In these patients, early surgical repair is indicated [5]. Good apposition is easily accomplished even with massive

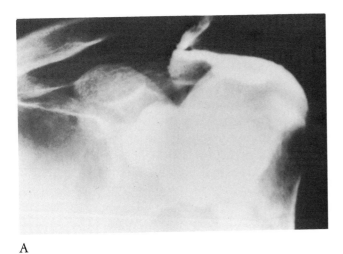

A

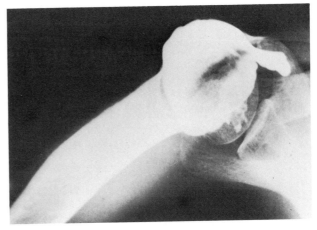

B

FIGURE 5-26. *Inadvertent injection of the subacromial-subdeltoid bursa.*

A. The internal rotation view might mistakenly be interpreted as an intracapsular injection showing a rotator cuff tear.

B. However, the axillary view shows there is no contrast in the joint. A repeat study was performed and the rotator cuff was normal.

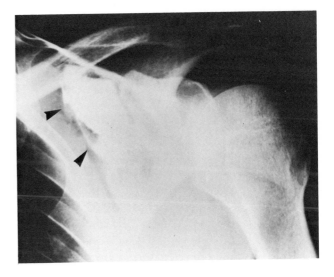

FIGURE 5-27. *Complete extravasation of contrast through the subscapularis bursa (black arrowheads).*

This patient had severe adhesive capsulitis, which made it impossible to perform an adequate shoulder arthrogram. Both single and double contrast techniques were attempted.

tears, because the tendons can be mobilized laterally and repaired primarily. The procedure may be combined with an acromioclavicular arthroplasty (acromioplasty and resection of the acromioclavicular ligament) if decompression of the subacromial space is necessary.

At the opposite end of the spectrum are the chronic rotator cuff lesions usually seen in elderly patients. Chronic tears are difficult to treat surgically owing to both the likelihood of coexisting medical conditions and the poor quality of the tendons to be repaired. Conservative therapy (physical rehabilitation, heat, anti-inflammatory agents) is indicated for a variable period of time depending on the patient's level of dysfunction and ultimate goals. Rehabilitation may produce improvement in some patients. If, however, conservative treatment fails to alleviate symptoms, then surgery may be necessary.

REFERENCES

1. Codman, E. A. *The Shoulder.* New York: G. Miller, 1934. Pp. 123–177.
2. Kessel, R. L. Injuries of the shoulder. In J. N. Wilson (Ed.), *Watson-Jones Fractures and Joint Injuries* (5th ed.). Edinburgh: Livingstone, 1976. Pp. 525–532.
3. McLaughlin, M. L. Rupture of the rotator cuff. *J. Bone Joint Surg.* 41(A):978, 1963.
4. Neer, C. S., II. Anterior acromioplasty for the chronic impingement syndrome in the shoulder. A preliminary report. *J. Bone Joint Surg.* 54(A):41, 1972.
5. Neer, C. S., II, and Welsh, P. The shoulder in sports. *Orthop. Clin. North Am.* 8:583, 1977.

SUGGESTED READING

Bakelim, G., and Pasila, M. Surgical treatment of ruptures of the rotator cuff tendon. *Acta Orthop. Scand.* 46:751, 1975.
Bateman, J. E. *The Shoulder and Neck* (2nd ed.). Philadelphia: Saunders, 1973. Pp. 140–141, 373, 440.
Bateman, J. E. Cuff tears in athletes. *Orthop. Clin. North Am.* 4:721, 1973.
Brewer, B. J. Aging of the rotator cuff. *Am. J. Sports Med.* 7:102, 1979.
Debeyre, D., Patie, D., and Elmelik, E. Repair of ruptures of the rotator cuffs of the shoulder with a note on advancement of the supraspinatus muscle. *J. Bone Joint Surg.* 47(B):36, 1965.
DePalma, A. F., Calley, G., and Bennett, G. A. Variational anatomy and degenerative lesions of the shoulder joint. Instructional Course Lectures. *Am. Acad. Orthop. Surg.* 6:255, 1949.

DePalma, A. F. *Surgery of the Shoulder* (2nd ed.). Philadelphia: Lippincott, 1973. Pp. 223–234.

Ghelman, B., and Goldman, A. B. The double contrast shoulder arthrogram. Evaluation of rotator cuff tears. *Radiology* 124:251, 1977.

Goldman, A. B., and Ghelman, B. The double contrast shoulder arthrogram. A review of 158 studies. *Radiology* 127:655, 1978.

Harrison, L., and McLaughlin, M. L. Rupture of the rotator cuff. *J. Bone Joint Surg.* 44(A):979, 1962.

Jackson, D. W. Chronic rotator cuff impingement in the throwing athlete. *Am. J. Sports Med.* 4:231, 1976.

Killoran, P. K., Marcove, R. C., and Freiberger, R. H. Shoulder arthrography. *A.J.R.* 103:658, 1968.

Lindblom, K., and Palmer, I. Ruptures of the tendon aponeurosis of the shoulder joint. The so-called supraspinatus rupture. *Acta Chir. Scand.* 82:133, 1939.

McLaughlin, M. L. Lesions of the musculo-tendinous cuff of the shoulder. *J. Bone Joint Surg.* 26:31, 1944.

Moseley, M. F. *Shoulder Lesions* (3rd ed.). Edinburgh: Livingstone, 1967. Pp. 60–87.

Nelson, C. L. The use of arthrography in athletic injuries of the shoulder. *Orthop. Clin. North Am.* 4:775, 1973.

Neviaser, J. S. Ruptures of the rotator cuff. *Clin. Orthop.* 3:92, 1954.

Neviaser, J. S. Ruptures of the rotator cuff of the shoulder. New concepts in the diagnosis and operative treatment of chronic ruptures. *Arch. Surg.* 102:483, 1971.

Neviaser, J. S. *Arthrography of the Shoulder. The Diagnosis and Management of the Lesions Visualized.* Springfield, Ill.: Thomas, 1975. Pp. 148–178.

Neviaser, J. S., Neviaser, R. J., and Neviaser, T. J. The repair of chronic massive ruptures of the rotator cuff of the shoulder by use of a freeze dried rotator cuff. *J. Bone Joint Surg.* 60(A):681, 1978.

Neviaser, R. J. Tears of the rotator cuff. *Orthop. Clin. North Am.* 11:295, 1980.

Nixon, J. E., and DiStephano, V. Ruptures of the rotator cuff. *Orthop. Clin. North Am.* 6:423, 1975.

Rowz, C. R. Ruptures of the rotator cuff. Selection of cases for conservative treatment. *Surg. Clin. North Am.* 43:1531, 1963.

Samilson, R. L., et al. Shoulder arthrography. *J.A.M.A.* 175:773, 1961.

Samilson, R. L., et al. Arthrography of the shoulder joint. *Clin. Orthop.* 20:21, 1961.

Samilson, R. L., and Binder, W. F. Symptomatic full thickness tears of the rotator cuff. An analysis of 292 shoulders in 276 patients. *Orthop. Clin. North Am.* 6:449, 1975.

Wolfgang, G. L. Surgical repair of tears of the rotator cuff of the shoulder. Factors influencing the result. *J. Bone Joint Surg.* 56(A):14, 1974.

Wolfgang, G. L. Rupture of musculotendinous cuff of the shoulder. *Clin. Orthop.* 134:230, 1978.

6 Abnormalities of the Tendon of the Long Head of the Biceps Brachii

The tendon of the long head of the biceps brachii can be evaluated on the double contrast shoulder arthrogram. With the double contrast technique, there is superior visualization of the insertion of the biceps tendon in the superior joint space and rarely does the tendon sheath fail to fill. Evaluation of the tendon of the long head of the biceps brachii has been noted to be difficult in series using the single contrast technique [7].

ANATOMY REVIEW

The tendon of the long head of the biceps brachii inserts proximal to the superior glenoid labrum, passes through the superior aspect of the joint capsule above the humeral head, and then enters the bicipital groove from above (Fig. 6-1). The roof of the groove is formed by the transverse humeral ligament and by the rotator cuff. Within the bicipital groove, and for a variable distance below it, the tendon is covered by a synovial lined capsular reflection or tendon sheath.

The tendon does not slide within the groove, but the humeral head at the groove glides on the tendon. The gliding motion helps the biceps muscle depress the humeral head when the arm is elevated.

PATHOPHYSIOLOGY

Close association with the rotator cuff, the coracoacromial arch, and the subacromial bursa renders the tendon of the long head of the biceps brachii susceptible to degenerative or traumatic ruptures, tenosynovitis, and subluxations or dislocations.

Ruptures of the tendon of the long head of the biceps are usually the result of a combination of attritional changes and trauma. Lesions of the rotator cuff and impingement syndromes expose the tendon of the long head of the biceps to chronic irritation and fraying. The pain that results from these chronic degenerative changes can mask the initial rupture, and subsequent episodes of trauma often go unnoticed. Over a period of time, the torn tendon can become fixed within the bicipital groove.

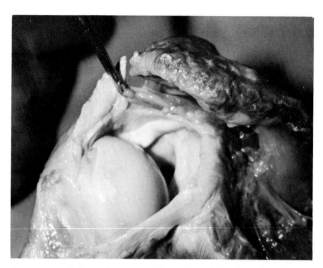

FIGURE 6-1. *Anatomy of tendon of the long head of the biceps brachii.*

The proximal portion of the tendon is intra-articular. It originates just above the superior glenoid labrum, passes through the top of the capsule, and then enters the groove between the greater and lesser tuberosities. Within the bicipital groove and for several centimeters below the groove the tendon is covered by a capsular reflection.

The etiology of tenosynovitis in the tendon of the long head of the biceps is variable. Predisposing factors include trauma, calcific peritendinitis, aging, and anatomic variations of the groove. A ridge in the proximal medial wall of the osseous intertubercular tunnel (the supratubercular ridge of Meyer), a shallow intertubercular groove, and a distorted groove secondary to fractures of the tuberosities have all been incriminated in tendinitis. Spurs adjacent to the tuberosities may also lead to inflammatory changes.

Medial subluxation or dislocation of the tendon of the long head of the biceps is frequently the result of forced external rotation of an abducted arm. Sometimes the tendon remains dislocated no matter what position the shoulder assumes, but in other cases, it returns to its normal osseous intertubercular groove on internal rotation. In some patients with complete dislocation, unroofing of the bicipital groove occurs as a result of disruption of the attachment of the supraspinatus tendon.

CLINICAL SIGNS AND SYMPTOMS

Physical examination of patients with abnormalities of the tendon of the long head of the biceps demonstrate anterior shoulder pain, crepitus, and in some cases, limitation of motion of the shoulder joint. Point tenderness in the region of the bicipital groove is extremely common. Tenosynovitis is particularly painful and may lead to adhesive capsulitis and the frozen shoulder syndrome [3, 4].

The two clinical tests indicative of biceps abnormalities, particularly in the region of the groove, are described by Yagerson and Speed. Yagerson's test is performed by supinating the forearm with the arm at the patient's side and the elbow flexed [2]. This motion causes pain if the tendon is damaged or inflamed. Speed's test is performed with the elbow extended and the hand supinated. The arm is lifted, and any pain in the region of the bicipital groove suggests instability [1].

In patients who have an acute tear of the biceps tendon, a large bump may be present along the anterior surface of the arm (Fig. 6-2). The presence and size of the soft tissue mass depends on the size of the muscle before its rupture and on the degree of retraction.

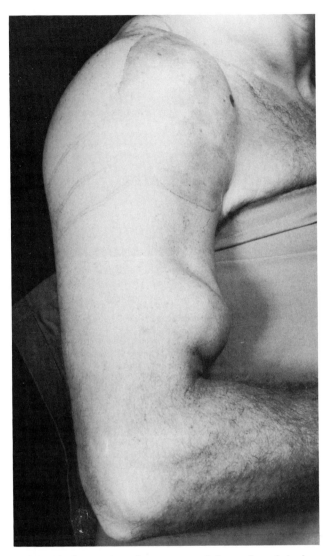

FIGURE 6-2. *Complete rupture of the tendon of the long head of the biceps.*
This athletic male presented with an abnormal soft tissue mass along the anterior aspect of the arm. The mass is formed by the detached muscle.
Sources: Goldman, A. B. and Ghelman, B. The double contrast shoulder arthrogram. A review of 158 studies. *Radiology* 127:655, 1978. With permission; Goldman, A. B. Double Contrast Shoulder Arthrography. In R. H. Freiberger and J. J. Kaye (Eds.), *Arthrography.* New York: Appleton-Century-Crofts, 1979.

PLAIN FILM FINDINGS

Abnormalities of the tendon of the long head of the biceps produce minimal and non-specific changes on plain films. The only specific finding is calcium deposits that are medial to the humeral head on internal rotation and lateral to the humeral head on external rotation, and indicate calcific peritendinitis (Fig. 6-3). However, there may be evidence of other conditions, which are associated with secondary damage to the biceps tendon, such as the shallow bicipital groove, post-traumatic deformities of the tuberosities, or signs of a chronic rotator cuff tear. There also may be evidence of sequelae of biceps abnormalities, particularly juxta-articular osteoporosis, suggestive of adhesive capsulitis.

ARTHROGRAPHIC ABNORMALITIES

On a double contrast study, the tendon of the long head of the biceps is coated with contrast and appears as a soft tissue density within the air-distended capsule and the tendon sheath (Fig. 6-4). On all views, the tendon and sheath should project between the tuberosities (Fig. 6-4). On a single contrast arthrogram, the tendon appears as a lucency within the contrast-filled sheath. The proximal intracapsular portion is usually covered by the dense positive contrast material (Fig. 6-5).

Complete Rupture

Complete rupture of the tendon of the long head of the biceps is diagnosed arthrographically by failure to visualize the shadow of the tendon either within the capsule or within the sheath (Figs. 6-6 to 6-9). There may also be some distortion and dilation of the sheath (Fig. 6-7). A complete rupture is best appreciated on the standing internal and external rotation views in which an air-contrast level can underscore the absence of the tendon (Fig. 6-6). If the tear is in the region of the tuberosities, it can also be demonstrated on the bicipital groove view (Fig. 6-6).

Tenosynovitis

Tenosynovitis of the tendon of the long head of the biceps is characterized arthrographically by an increase in the width of the tendon and a loss of the sharp, smooth margin of the sheath, indicative of edema and adhesions (Figs. 6-10, 6-11).

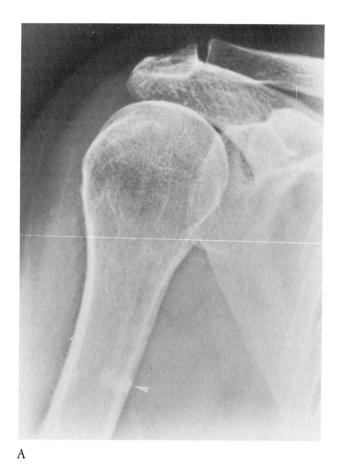

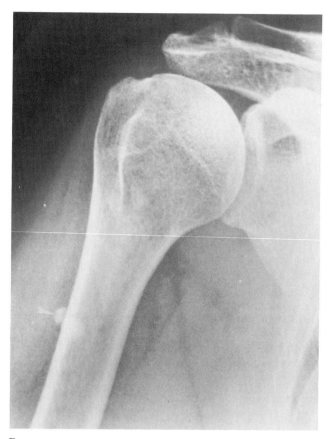

A

B

FIGURE 6-3. *Calcific tendinitis of the long head of the biceps.*

A. On the internal rotation view calcium is noted below the tuberosities and medial to the humeral shaft (white arrowhead).

B. On the external rotation view the calcific deposit rotates lateral to the humeral shaft (white arrowhead). Calcification in the bursae, the major differential diagnosis, would also be below the tuberosities. However, unlike biceps tendinitis, the densities would remain lateral to the humeral head on both views.

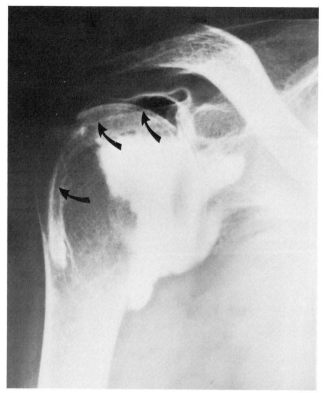

A

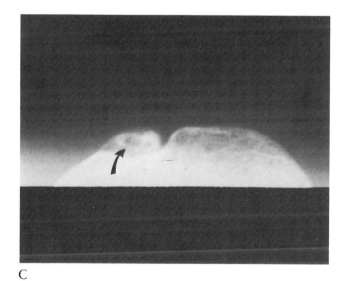

C

B

FIGURE 6-4. *Normal appearance of the tendon of the long head of the biceps on a double contrast arthrogram.*

On the external rotation, A, axillary, B, and bicipital groove, C, views, the tendon appears as a soft tissue density within the superior capsule and within the tendon sheath (curved black arrows). On all projections, the tendon is seen within the sheath and both tendon and sheath are between the tuberosities.

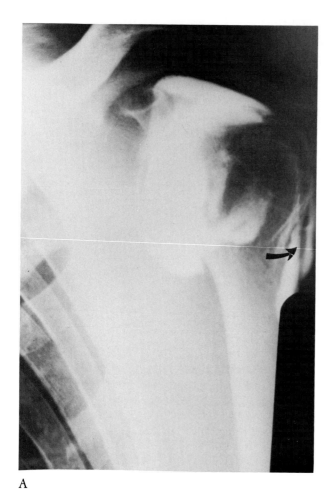

A

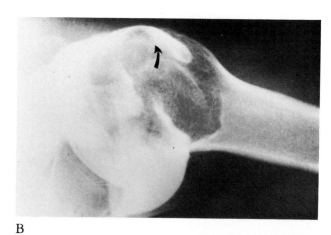

B

C

FIGURE 6-5. *Normal appearance of the tendon of the long head of the biceps on a single contrast arthrogram.*

On the external rotation, A, axillary, B, and bicipital groove, C, views, the tendon appears as a lucency within the sheath (curved black arrows). The intracapsular portion of the tendon is obscured by the dense positive contrast within the superior portion of the capsule.

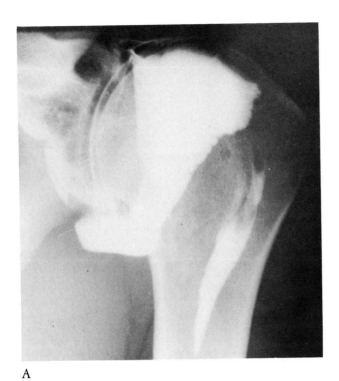

A

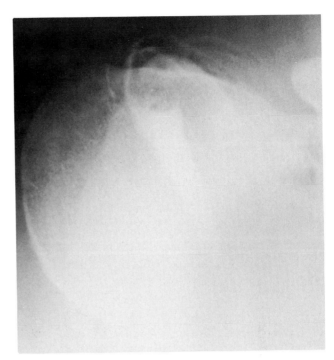

B

FIGURE 6-6. *Complete rupture of the tendon of the long head of the biceps.*

The external rotation, A, and bicipital groove, B, views show an air contrast level within the sheath but the soft tissue shadow of the tendon is absent.

Sources: Goldman, A. B. and Ghelman, B. The double contrast shoulder arthrogram. A review of 158 studies. *Radiology* 127:655, 1978. With permission; Goldman, A. B. Double Contrast Shoulder Arthrography. In R. H. Freiberger and J. J. Kaye (Eds.), *Arthrography.* New York: Appleton-Century-Crofts, 1979. P. 182.

90

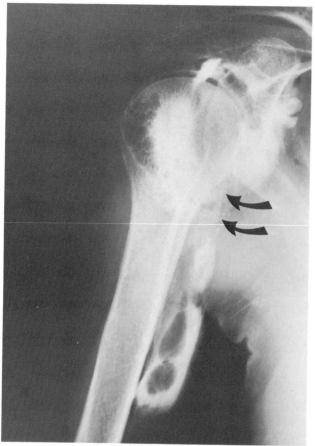

A

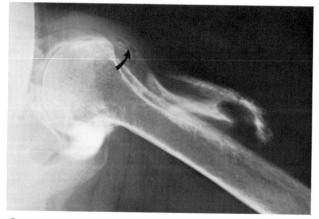

C

B

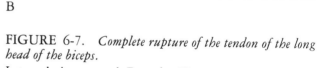

FIGURE 6-7. *Complete rupture of the tendon of the long head of the biceps.*

Internal, A, external, B, and axillary, C, views show collapse of the sheath and no shadow of the tendon— just distal to the tuberosities (curved black arrows). Below the area of the tear the sheath and tendon are irregular and distorted.

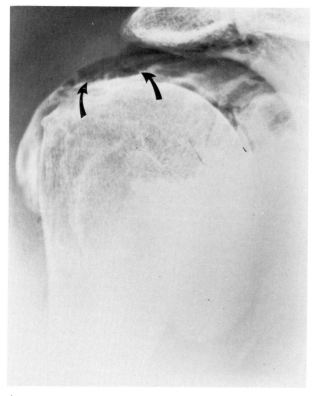

A

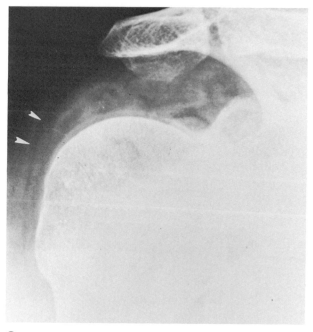

C

B

FIGURE 6-8. *Complete rupture of the tendon of the long head of the biceps.*

A. The external rotation view demonstrates an abnormal interruption of the soft tissue shadow of the tendon just proximal to the tuberosities (curved black arrows).

B. The axillary view shows an empty air-filled sheath between the tuberosities (curved arrows).

C. The internal rotation view demonstrates a coexisting rotator cuff tear with air in the subacromial-subdeltoid bursa (white arrowheads).

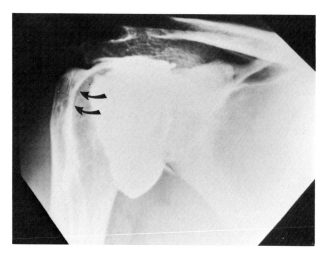

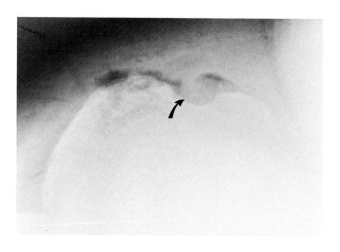

FIGURE 6-9. *Complete rupture of the tendon of long head of the biceps diagnosed on single contrast study.*
The sheath between and below the tuberosities is empty and collapsed (curved black arrows). No lucent shadow of the tendon is seen in that segment.

FIGURE 6-10. *Biceps tendinitis.*
The soft tissue shadow of the tendon fills the groove (curved black arrow). Its margin is also noted to be irregular.

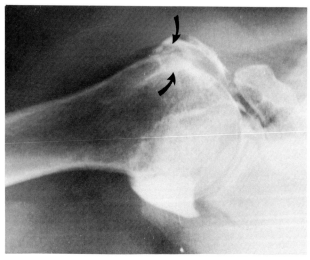

A

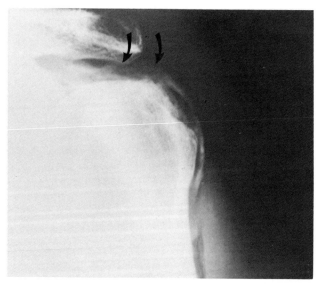

B

FIGURE 6-11. *Biceps tendinitis.*
A. The axillary view shows swelling of the tendon with its shadow extending beyond the tuberosities (curved black arrows).
B. The external rotation view reveals irregularity of the contour of the tendon (curved black arrows).

Medial Dislocation and/or Subluxation

Medial dislocation or subluxation of the tendon of the long head of the biceps is most easily identified on the bicipital groove and axillary views (Fig. 6-12). On the bicipital groove view, the osseous tunnel is seen en face and if there is a dislocation, the groove is empty and the soft tissue shadow of the tendon, surrounded by its sheath, is seen medial to the tuberosities (Fig. 6-12). On the axillary view, the bicipital groove is seen in profile and if there is a dislocation, the tendon projects anterior to the tuberosities (Fig. 6-12B).

However, in some patients the dislocation is position dependent and the diagnosis can be established only with serial internal and external rotation views (Fig. 6-13). In these patients, the tendon assumes its normal position on the internal rotation, axillary, and bicipital groove views. It is only on the external rotation view that the tendon does not project between the tuberosities (Fig. 6-12C). Care must be taken to insure that the shoulder is in maximal external rotation to prevent false negatives. Preferably, a second set of films should be performed to confirm the diagnosis.

In some individuals, particularly those with shallow bicipital grooves, the tendon may not rest in the center of the tunnel, but may sit adjacent to, or actually on, the lesser tuberosity (Fig. 6-14). The clinical significance of subluxation of the tendon of the long head of the biceps has not been established.

CAUSES FOR MISINTERPRETATION

False-positive studies can result from mistaking leakage of contrast from the distal end of the biceps tendon sheath for an abnormality of the tendon (Fig. 6-15). The integrity of the capsular reflection is unrelated to the status of the tendon. The sheath is a normal weak point in the joint capsule, and leakage is related to mechanical factors, including the capacity of the capsule, the volume of contrast injected, and the amount of intra-articular pressure generated during exercise. Another pitfall is extreme swelling of the tendon that makes it project beyond the margin of the groove (Fig. 6-11A). This appearance can result in an incorrect diagnosis of dislocation.

False-negative studies are by far a greater problem than false-positive studies in the evaluation of the tendon of the long head of the biceps. In some

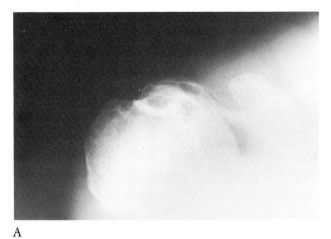

A

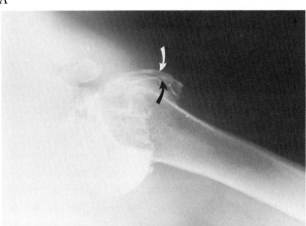

B

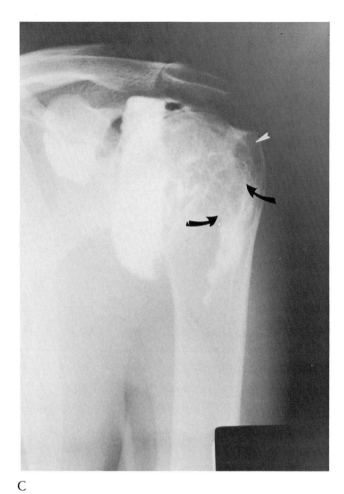

C

FIGURE 6-12.   *Medial dislocation of the tendon of the long head of the biceps.*

A. The bicipital groove view reveals an empty osseous tunnel.

B. The axillary view demonstrates that the sheath is filled and the tendon is within the sheath, but both are anterior to the tuberosities (curved arrows).

C. The external rotation view shows scalloping of the sheath and demonstrates the tendon (curved black arrows) medial to the groove (white arrowhead).

Sources: Goldman, A. B. and Ghelman, B. The double contrast shoulder arthrogram. A review of 158 studies. *Radiology* 127:655, 1978. With permission; Goldman, A. B. Double Contrast Shoulder Arthrography. In R. H. Freiberger and J. J. Kaye (Eds.), *Arthrography.* New York: Appleton-Century-Crofts, 1979. P. 185.

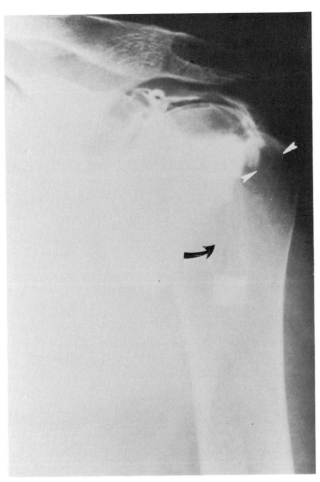

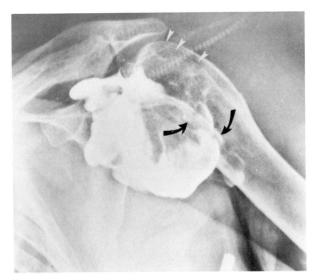

FIGURE 6-13. *Two cases of medial dislocation of the tendon at the long head of the biceps seen only on serial external rotation views.*

A. A double contrast study shows the tendon and sheath (curved black arrow) projected medial to the osseous groove (white arrowheads).

B. A single contrast study reveals the tendon and its irregular sheath (curved black arrows) projected medial to the osseous bicipital groove (white arrowheads).

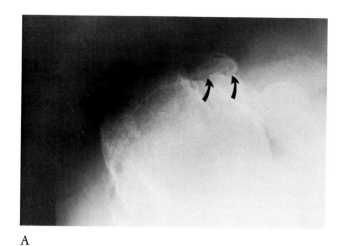

A

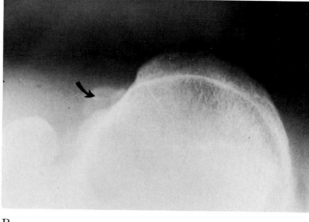

B

FIGURE 6-14. *Medial subluxation of the tendon of the long head of the biceps.*

A. A patient with the tendon sitting on the lesser tuberosity (curved black arrows). The tendon is also swollen and irregular.

B. A second patient has a shallow bicipital groove and eccentrically seated tendon (curved black arrow).

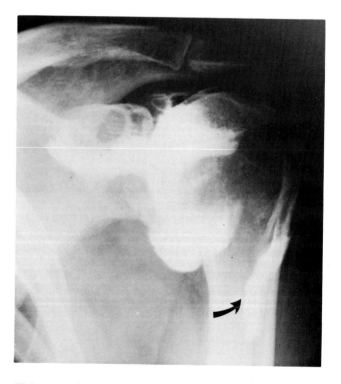

FIGURE 6-15. *Extravasation of contrast from distal end of sheath (curved black arrow).*

This leakage is unrelated to abnormalities of the tendon. It results either from decreased volume of the capsule or excessive distention of the capsule.

instances there is failure to fill the synovial-lined sheath. Although this failure may indicate pathology of the tendon with swelling and adhesions, it can also indicate adhesive capsulitis, and is therefore a nonspecific finding. Another cause for false-negative studies of the tendon of the long head of the biceps is a coexisting rotator cuff tear. Air and contrast within the subacromial-subdeltoid bursa obscure the biceps tendon and in some cases make evaluation extremely difficult. A rupture of the tendon may occur below the level of the synovial-lined sheath and therefore cannot be seen on the arthrogram.

TREATMENT

Initial treatment of inflammatory lesions of the long head of the biceps tendon is conservative and includes rest, heat, and anti-inflammatory agents, followed by an active stretching program. Steroid injections may be beneficial in cases of persistent tenosynovitis. If symptoms persist, surgery may be indicated. The surgery of inflammatory lesions of the long head of the biceps tendon consists of a tenodesis procedure, whereby the tendon is permanently anchored into the bicipital groove (Hitchcock Procedure) or is transposed to the coronoid process. Because additional pathology is often found at the time of surgery, Dines et al. note that care must be taken to thoroughly explore the rotator cuff, the undersurface of the acromioclavicular joint, and the stability of the glenohumeral joint [6].

In cases of medial dislocation of the tendon of the long head of the biceps, surgery is usually indicated, since conservative therapy is of little benefit. Tenodesis is carried out and, in cases of documented instability of the tendon, the results are usually good.

Nontraumatic or degenerative ruptures of the long head of the biceps tendon generally occur as the result of an impingement syndrome. These ruptures are relatively asymptomatic initially, but may subsequently be associated with the pain of an impingement process or rotator cuff tear. In patients under forty-five years of age, surgery is recommended and should include an exploration of the subacromial space and tenodesis of the biceps tendon. In the older individual, surgery may be deferred as weakness of elbow flexion is not a significant problem [5].

REFERENCES

1. Abbott, L. E., Saunders, B. De C. M. Acute traumatic dislocation of the tendon of the long head of biceps brachii. A report of six cases with operative findings. *Surgery* 6:817, 1939.
2. Bateman, J. E. *The Shoulder and Neck.* Philadelphia: Saunders, 1978. Pp. 329–338.
3. Crenshaw, A. M. and Kilgore, W. E. Surgical treatment of bicipital tenosynovitis. *J. Bone Joint Surg.* 48(A):1496, 1966.
4. DePalma, A. F. Frozen shoulder. *Am. Acad. Orthop. Surg.* Instructional Course Lectures. 9:313, 1952.
5. DePalma, A. F. Surgery of the Shoulder (2nd ed.). Philadelphia: Lippincott, 1973. Pp. 468–470.
6. Dines, D. M., Warren, R., and Inglis, A. E. The surgical treatment of lesions of the long head of the biceps. *Clin. Orthop.* 164:165–171, 1982.
7. Nelson, D. H. Arthrography of the shoulder. *Br. J. Radiol.* 25:134, 1952.

SUGGESTED READING

Booth, R. E., Jr., and Marvel, J. P., Jr. Differential diagnosis of shoulder pain. *Orthop. Clin. North Am.* 6:353, 1975.

Codman, E. A. *The Shoulder.* New York: Miller, 1934. Pp. 501–502.

Goldman, A. B., and Ghelman, B. The double contrast shoulder arthrogram. A review of 158 studies. *Radiology* 127:655, 1978.

Hitchcock, H. M., and Bechtol, C. O. Painful shoulders, observations on the role of the tendon of the long head of the biceps brachii in its causation. *J. Bone Joint Surg.* 30(A):263, 1948.

Lippman, R. K. Frozen shoulder; periarthritis; bicipital tenosynovitis. *Arch. Surg.* 47:283, 1943.

Meyer, A. W. Unrecognized occupational destruction of the tendon of the long head of the biceps brachii. *Arch. Surg.* 2:139, 1921.

Meyer, A. W. Spontaneous dislocation of the long head of the biceps brachii. Report of four cases. *Arch. Surg.* 13:109, 1926.

Meyer, A. W. Chronic functional lesions of the shoulder. *Arch. Surg.* 35:646, 1937.

Mitchcoel, M. M., and Bechtol, C. O. Painful shoulder. *J. Bone Joint Surg.* 30(A):263, 1948.

Neer, C. S., II. Anterior acromioplasty for chronic impingement syndrome of the shoulder. *J. Bone Joint Surg.* 54(A):41, 1972.

Neer, C. S., II, and Welsh, R. P. The shoulder in sports. *Orthop. Clin. North Am.* 8:583, 1977.

Neviaser, R. J. Lesions of the biceps and tendinitis of the shoulder. *Orthop. Clin. North Am.* 2:343, 1980.

O'Donoghue, D. H. Subluxing biceps tendon in the athlete. *J. Sports Med.* 1:20, 1973.

Pasteur, F. Le teno-bursite bicipitale. *J. Radiol. Electro.* 16:419, 1932.

Samilson, R. L., Raphael, R. L., Post, L., et al. Shoulder arthrography. *J.A.M.A.* 179:773, 1961.

Schrager, V. C. Tenosynovitis of the long head of the biceps humeri. *Surg. Gynecol. Obstet.* 66:785, 1938.

7

Postdislocation Abnormalities of the Articular Cartilages of the Humerus and Glenoid

The most frequent cartilage abnormalities of the shoulder are those related to previous dislocations of the humeral head. Shoulder dislocations were described by Hippocrates in 460 B.C. He also described techniques for reducing the dislocation and for preventing its recurrence. His recommendation was to use a burning poker to produce adhesions in the soft tissues surrounding the joint, warning surgeons to avoid the great vessels and nerves in the area. Current surgical management still relies on Hippocrates' principles: achieving stability of the joint and avoiding the adjacent neurovascular structures.

ANATOMY REVIEW

The high frequency of dislocations of the shoulder is due in part to the anatomy of the glenohumeral joint. The shoulder has (1) the large humeral head articulating with a relatively small, shallow glenoid fossa (Fig. 7-1) and (2) a loose, capsular support resulting in poor osseous stability with stress on the surrounding soft tissue structures. If the humeral head dislocates anteriorly, its posterior aspect impinges upon the anteroinferior aspect of the glenoid, causing compression fractures of the superolateral aspect of the humeral head and avulsions of the anterior inferior glenoid labrum and/or articular cartilage. If the humeral head dislocates posteriorly, the anteromedial aspect of the humeral head hits the posterior glenoid labrum, resulting in fractures and the subscapularis tendon becoming stretched across the anterior glenoid labrum.

PATHOPHYSIOLOGY

Traumatic dislocations of the shoulder can be classified according to the abnormal position of the humeral head following injury. The major categories are anterior, posterior, and multidirectional.

Anterior Dislocations and Subluxations

Anterior dislocations are subdivided into subcoracoid, inferior (subglenoid), and subclavicular

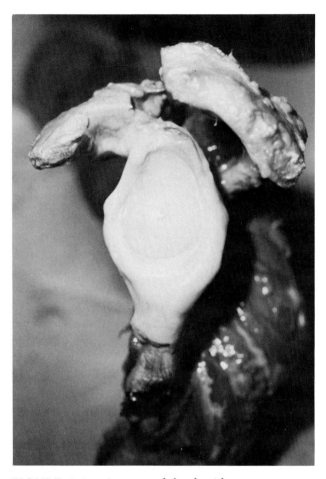

FIGURE 7-1. *Anatomy of the glenoid.*
The glenoid is a small shallow fossa that contains the much larger humeral head. Dislocations of the humeral head are therefore not infrequent and may result in fractures of the glenoid rim. The site of the glenoid fracture or fractures reflects the direction of the dislocation.

categories based on the position of the humeral head following injury.

Anterior subcoracoid dislocations comprise approximately 90 percent of all anterior derangements of the glenohumeral joint. They usually occur as the result of an indirect force with external rotation applied to an abducted arm. Less commonly, a subcoracoid dislocation results from a direct posterior blow to the shoulder. The inferior (subglenoid) anterior dislocations are less common than the subcoracoid type. The rare *luxatio erecta* dislocation is included in this category. The anterior inferior glenohumeral dislocations result from forced hyperabduction of the humerus. The neck of the humerus impinges on the acromion and levers the head of the humerus out of the glenoid cavity. The inferiorly displaced humeral head tears the inferior capsule and the downward-directed humeral head locks below the inferior lip of the glenoid. The shaft of the humerus can point straight up. Inferior dislocations often have associated osteochondral and soft tissue complications, including fractures of the acromion, the inferior glenoid rim, and the greater tuberosity; brachial plexus injuries; and tears of the rotator cuff. The subclavicular and intrathoracic anterior glenohumeral dislocations are least common and occur as the result of a direct lateral blow accompanied by severe external rotation of the shoulder and abduction of the humerus. These injuries are extremely serious and can be accompanied by significant damage to the intrathoracic structures.

Traumatic anterior dislocations frequently recur, and a combination of predisposing factors are probably responsible. Many of the implicated lesions are as yet highly controversial. First, the age of the patient is influential. Patients under the age of 20 have a recurrence rate of over 90 percent, whereas patients over the age of 40 have a recurrence rate of only 15 percent [16, 17, 18, 19]. Second, a coexisting fracture of the proximal humerus appears to reduce the incidence of a second dislocation. A third, and less well established variable, is generalized ligamentous laxity. In a review of recurrent dislocations reported by Kinnett et al. [8], soft tissue laxity was noted to be a significant factor in the recurrence of dislocations in patients over the age of 40. Fourth, damage to the anterior inferior glenoid labrum (the Bankart deformity [1, 2] or a compression fracture of the posterior superior aspect of the humeral head (the

Hill-Sachs lesion) are postulated as factors leading to repetitive dislocations. Fifth, damage to the attachment of the capsule of the glenoid is also implicated in recurrent dislocations [13, 14, 22]. In a study published by Tijmes [22], leakage of contrast material outside of the confines of the joint capsule could be observed in the first 48 hours following injury. However, leakage occurred in only 48 percent of the patients, suggesting that the humeral head does not invariably tear the capsule. It is the contention of investigators, including Tullos [22] and Reeves [13, 14], that in many cases, the humeral head dissects below the glenoid periosteum, creating a cavity that communicates with the joint capsule. This abnormal space results in an effective enlargement of the anterior capsule. The sixth factor in recurrent dislocations—preexisting laxity of the subscapularis muscle or tendon—is a highly controversial topic. Symeonides [21] postulates that this structure exerts a major influence on the stability of the glenohumeral joint. However, Turkel et al. [23] and others have found that the inferior glenohumeral ligament plays a more significant role than the subscapularis.

Related to anterior dislocation is recurrent subluxation of the glenohumeral joint, often found in athletes who engage in sports that stress the glenohumeral joint: football, swimming, basketball, and tennis. In all these activities, the inferior glenohumeral ligament is subjected to either sudden blows or repeated stress. In some individuals, subluxation may progress to dislocation.

Posterior Dislocations, Posterior Subluxations, and Multidirectional Dislocators

Posterior dislocations are rare. The most common mechanism involves a combination of internal rotation of the shoulder and adduction and flexion of the humerus. Less frequently, posterior glenohumeral dislocations result from a fall on an outstretched hand or a grand mal seizure when the strong internal rotators overcome the weaker external rotators of the shoulder. It rarely results from a forceful direct blow to the anterior aspect of the shoulder.

Recurrent posterior subluxations can occur, and are most commonly seen in athletes who participate in throwing sports where the posterior inferior rim of the glenoid is stretched during the "follow-through" phase.

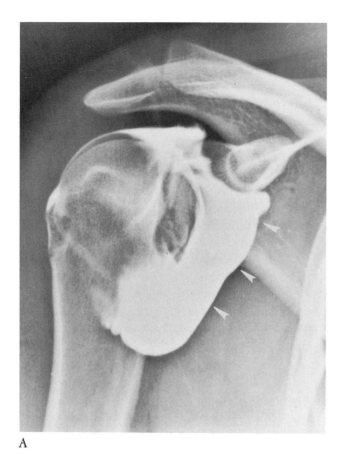

A

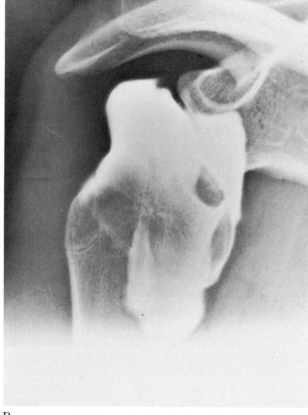

B

FIGURE 7-2. *Voluntary anterior dislocation of the shoulder.*

A. A routine internal rotation view from a single contrast arthrogram reveals an enlarged medial capsule, with loss of the normal indentation between the axillary recess and subscapularis bursa (white arrowheads) but the humeral head is located.

B. On request the patient dislocated her humeral head downward, medial, and anterior.

Inferior multidirectional instability of the shoulder, as described by Neer and Foster [11], combines anterior and posterior displacement of the humerus. These patients may dislocate in one direction and subluxate in the other, or they may dislocate in both directions. Many of these patients are "loose jointed," but most come to medical attention because of a significant injury.

There is another distinct group of patients who can voluntarily dislocate their glenohumeral joints in one or more directions (Fig. 7-2). There is a high association between voluntary dislocators and psychiatric disturbances. However, in patients with or without supratentorial problems, this voluntary "trick" may occasionally progress to an involuntary permanent injury and require treatment.

CLINICAL FINDINGS

Anterior Dislocations and Subluxations

The patient with an acute traumatic anterior dislocation presents with severe pain, a "squared off" appearance to the shoulder (due to absence of the normal subacromial roundness), prominence of the coracoid process, and an abnormal fullness in front of the coracoid.

A competitive athlete with recurrent anterior subluxations is a more difficult diagnostic problem: he or she usually presents with a sensation of "the shoulder going out" followed by aching pain. Snapping and clicking are also common complaints. Clinical diagnosis depends on careful repeated examination and on a relaxed patient.

Posterior Dislocations, Posterior Subluxations, and Multidirectional Dislocators

Patients with acute posterior dislocation of the humeral head present with severe pain. The affected limb is held in adduction and internal rotation. Physical examination reveals an inability to externally rotate the shoulder and abduct the humerus. In thin individuals, abnormal anterior flattening, and/or an abnormal posterior prominence may be observed.

Patients with repeated posterior subluxations or multidirectional instability present with vague diffuse shoulder pain. The affected shoulder may sag inferiorly with stress. As with anterior subluxations, careful examination of a relaxed shoulder (which may require general anesthesia) can indicate the diagnosis.

PLAIN FILM FINDINGS
Anterior Dislocations and Subluxations

The diagnosis of an acute anterior glenohumeral dislocation is usually established on the plain antero-posterior films. The roentgen appearance depends on the position of the humeral head in relation to the anatomic landmarks of the scapula. In the most frequent type of dislocation, the subcoracoid, the humeral head is displaced downward anterior and medial to the glenoid (Fig. 7-3). The humeral head then rests below the coracoid process (Fig. 7-3). In the less frequent subglenoid dislocation, there is no medial component and the head is shifted downward and anteriorly, resting immediately below the glenoid. The humeral shaft can be fixed in an upward direction (Fig. 7-4). In the rare subclavicular type of dislocation, the plain film is characterized by a medial and intrathoracic position of the humeral head. Although the diagnosis is usually evident on routine antero-posterior films, transscapular, transthoracic, or axillary views may be of help in confirming the diagnosis and direction of the dislocation (Fig. 7-3). The transscapular view (Fig. 7-3) is usually preferable because it is easier to interpret than the transthoracic projection, on which overlap of other structures can be confusing [20]. The transscapular view has also been referred to as the Y view of the scapula and is a 60° anterior oblique of the injured shoulder [20]. The body of the scapula forms the vertical portion of the Y, the coracoid process is the anterior arm of the Y, and the acromion process is the posterior arm of the Y. The glenoid appears as a ring at the intersection of these three lines (Fig. 7-3C). In a normal individual the center of the humeral head is over the center of the glenoid. Axillary views (Figs. 7-3, 7-4) are frequently difficult to obtain in the emergency room since, unlike the other two projections, they require moving the injured extremity and movement is frequently impossible because of pain and spasm.

Immediately following closed reduction, the transscapular view can confirm the position of the humeral head in the glenoid [20]. On a postreduction internal rotation view, it is possible to determine the presence and extent of compression fractures of the posterior lateral aspect of the humeral head (the Hill-Sachs deformity) (Fig. 7-5A). A forced external rotation view is not advisable since it can result in a redislocation of the shoulder. However, a modified view with the arm in neutral

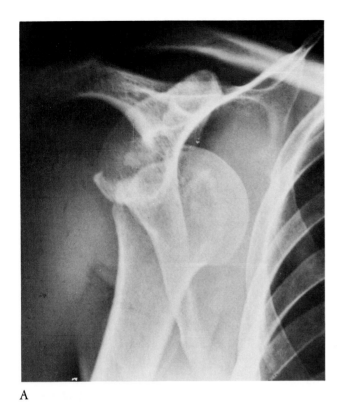

A

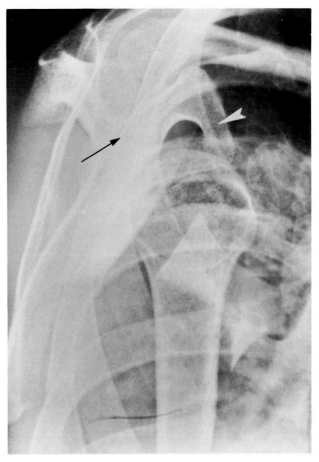

B

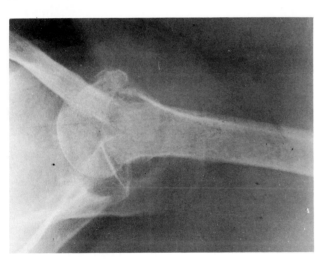

C

FIGURE 7-3.   *Subcoracoid anterior dislocation.*
A. On the antero-posterior view the humeral head is displaced inferior and medial to the glenoid.
B. The transscapular view shows the humeral head to be anterior to the glenoid (black arrow) and below the coracoid (white arrowhead).
C. Axillary view showing the back of the humeral head impinging on the front of the glenoid.

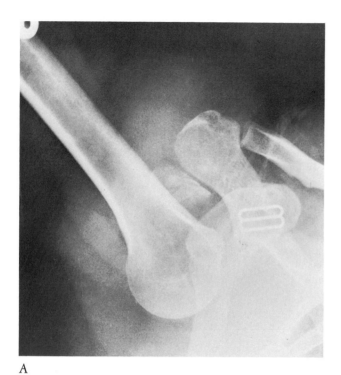

A

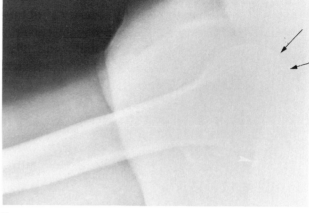

B

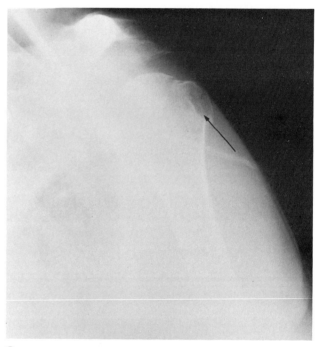

C

FIGURE 7-4. *Subglenoid (luxatio erecta) dislocation.*

A. The antero-posterior view demonstrates the shaft of the humerus impinging on the acromion process and levering the humeral head inferior to the glenoid. The shaft of the humerus points straight up. A fracture fragment is noted between the humeral shaft and acromion.

B. An axillary view of limited quality was obtained and confirmed that the articular surface of the humeral head (black arrows) was anterior to the glenoid (white arrowheads).

C. A postreduction antero-posterior oblique view with mild external rotation confirms the presence of a fracture of the greater tuberosity (black arrow).

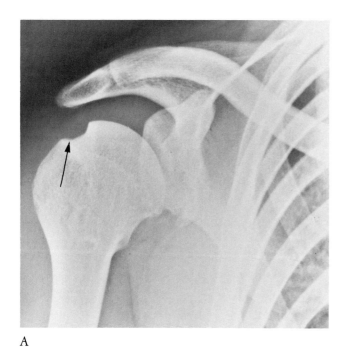

A

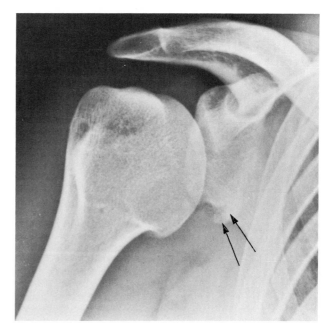

B

FIGURE 7-5. *Postdislocation compression fractures.*

A. The internal rotation view best shows the Hill-Sachs defect, which is a compression deformity of the posterior, superior, lateral aspect of the humeral head (black arrow).

B. The external rotation view demonstrates an avulsion of the articular cortex of the inferior glenoid (black arrows) referred to as an osseous Bankart defect.

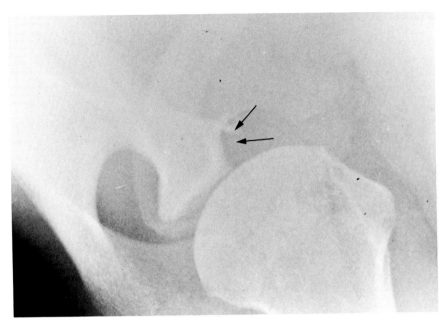

A

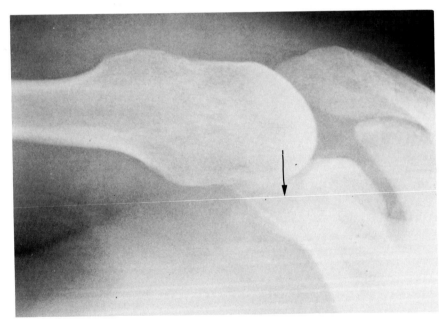

B

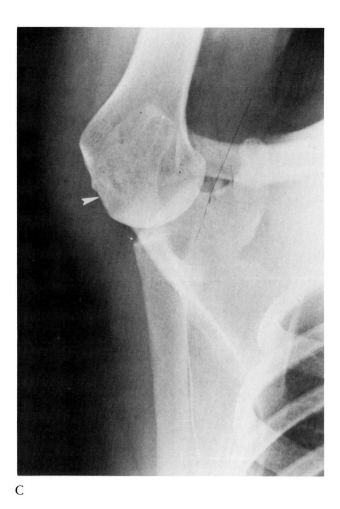

C

FIGURE 7-6. *Instability series.*
The prone axillary view, A, and Didiee view, B, show
an osseous Bankart defect (black arrows). The Stryker
view, C, reveals slight flattening of the posterior cortex
of the humeral head (white arrowhead). The small detached fragment seen on the prone axillary view, A,
may either be a chip fracture or small area of myositis
ossificans.

rotation and the shoulder obliqued 25° posteriorly
can demonstrate the inferior aspect of the glenoid
and make it possible to evaluate the presence and
extent of compression fractures of the osseous
glenoid (the Bankart defect, Fig. 7-5B). The lesion
originally described by Bankart [2] was limited to
the anterior inferior glenoid labrum and could not
be seen on plain films. However, his name is now
applied to all injuries of the osseous or cartilaginous inferior glenoid that follow an anterior dislocation. The oblique antero-posterior view also permits evaluation of the tuberosities which may not
be adequately seen with the shoulder dislocated
(Fig. 7-4C). Displaced fractures of the tuberosities
and detachment of the rotator cuff are occasionally
sequelae of an anterior dislocation.

In patients with a history of anterior subluxations of the shoulder or in patients with a history
of a previously treated dislocation, the additional
studies in the "instability series" can demonstrate
small compression defects not seen on the routine
views (Fig. 7-6). Specifically, the additional views
include the West Point prone axillary view [10],
the Stryker or "notch" view [15], and the Didiee
view [15] (Fig. 7-6).

Posterior Dislocations and Subluxations
The diagnosis of an acute or chronic posterior dislocation of the humeral head is difficult to establish
on standard internal and external rotation projections as the findings are subtle and may be easily
missed. Findings that indicate a possible posterior
displacement of the humeral head include the inability to externally rotate the shoulder (Figs. 7-7,
7-8), a minimal upward displacement of the humeral head (Figs. 7-7, 7-8), or a compression deformity of the medial aspect of the humeral head
referred to as the "trough" sign [5] (Fig. 7-7). If
the humeral head is wedged behind the glenoid,
there is an abnormal overlap of the humerus and
the anterior wall of the glenoid (Fig. 7-8A). However, if the humeral head is only partially displaced
from the glenoid cavity, there is instead an abnormal increase in the distance between the anterior
walls of the glenoid and the medial aspect of the
humeral head (Fig. 7-7). Therefore, depending on
the degree of displacement of the humeral head,
the normal overlap with the glenoid may be decreased or increased.

If the internal and external rotation views are
even slightly suspicious, other plain film studies

110

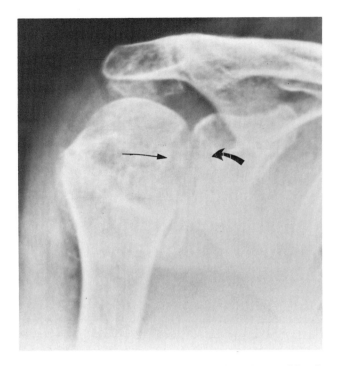

FIGURE 7-7. *Posterior dislocation of the humeral head.*
The antero-posterior view reveals an inability to coop-
erate for the internal and external rotation view,
minimal upward displacement of the humeral head,
and a medial compression fracture of the humeral
head. In this case, the distance between the cortex of
the humeral head (straight black arrow) and the cortex
of the anterior glenoid (curved black arrow) is increased.

should be performed to confirm or exclude the
diagnosis. Under fluoroscopic control, an antero-
posterior view can be obtained with the patient
obliqued posteriorly 25° to view the joint in tangent (Fig. 7-8A). On this projection, the glenoid
should appear as a straight line with both the anterior and posterior walls superimposed. On the
normal oblique antero-posterior view, there is no
overlap between the humeral head and the scapula.
In patients with a posterior dislocation, there is an
overlap between the two bones (Fig. 7-8A). Axillary (Fig. 7-8B), transscapular (Fig. 7-8C, and
transthoracic (Fig. 7-8D) views also help demonstrate posterior displacements of the humeral
head. On the transscapular view (Fig. 7-8C) the
glenoid is seen en face, and on the axillary and
transthoracic views it is seen in profile (Fig. 7-
8B, D). On all views the relationship between the
two articular surfaces can be easily appreciated. In
the acutely injured patient, the transscapular view
is easier to obtain than the axillary view since the
patient need not move the injured extremity.

ARTHROGRAPHIC FINDINGS

There are several indications for arthrography in
patients with a history of glenohumeral dislocation. First, in cases in which the history is
equivocal, the arthrogram may provide evidence of
a dislocation or subluxation. Second, the distribution of secondary osteocartilaginous abnormalities
can confirm the direction of the dislocation. Third,
in patients with a known dislocation, the decision
for surgical intervention may depend on the presence and extent of secondary capsular and osteocartilaginous abnormalities. Fourth, persistent
pain following reduction of a dislocation can result
from a coexisting rotator cuff tear or from loose
osteocartilaginous fragments, which can be identified arthrographically.

Anterior Dislocations and Subluxations

Documentation of a previous anterior dislocation
of the glenohumeral joint, evaluation of the direction and/or directions of the dislocation, and evaluation of the extent of the post-traumatic damage
depend on identifying secondary capsular and osteocartilaginous deformities. Figure 7-9 reviews
the smooth appearance of the medial joint capsule,
with a normal indentation between the axillary recess and subscapularis bursa.

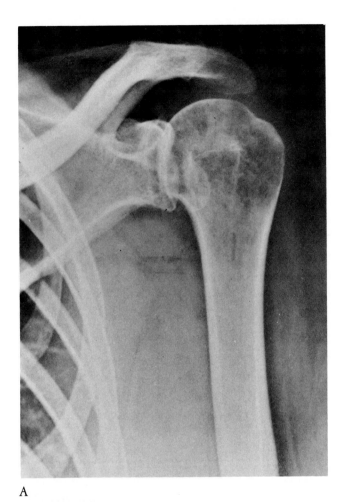

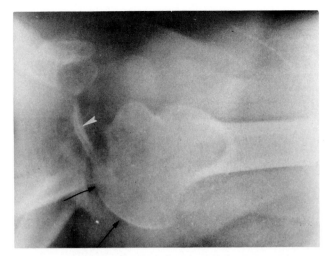

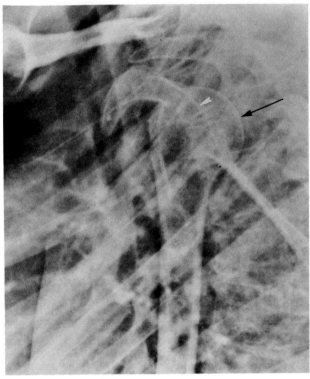

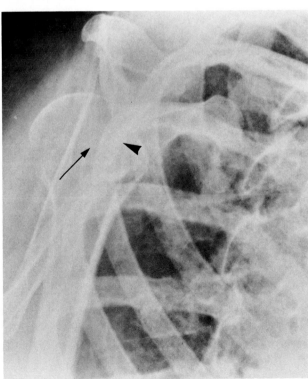

A

B

C

D

FIGURE 7-8. *Posterior dislocation of the humeral head.*

A. An antero-posterior view of the shoulder with the patient obliqued 25° posteriorly so that the glenoid appears as a straight line shows an abnormal overlap between the humeral head and glenoid. The humeral head is also slightly high in position.

B. The axillary view demonstrates the articular surface of the humerus (black arrows) to be behind the articular surface of the glenoid (white arrowhead).

C. The transscapular view reveals the center of the humeral head (arrow) to be behind the center of the glenoid (arrowhead).

D. The transthoracic view demonstrates the articular surface of the humeral head (black arrow) to be posterior to the cortex of the glenoid (white arrowhead).

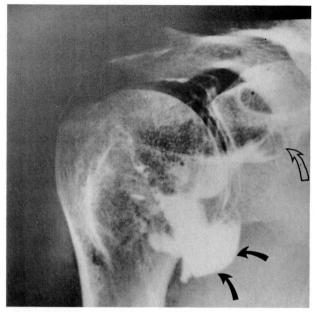

A

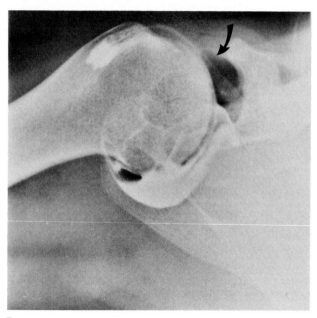

B

FIGURE 7-9. *Normal capsule.*

A. The external rotation view reveals a smooth capsular margin. Its medial aspect has the appearance of a figure "3," with a normal indentation between the axillary recess (curved black arrows) and subscapularis bursa (hollow black arrow). Extravasation of contrast can occur from the subscapularis bursa, which is a normal weak point in the joint capsule, but not from the axillary recess or inferomedial portion of the capsule.

B. The axillary view shows the normal capacity of the anterior capsule when outlined by air (curved black arrow).

Capsular abnormalities can be diagnosed on both single and double contrast arthrograms. If the contrast study is performed within 48 hours of injury, leakage of contrast material can frequently be demonstrated outside of the confines of the medial or inferior joint capsule [9, 13, 14, 22] (Figs. 7-10, 7-11). After 48 hours, leakage is almost never observed, since the capsule becomes watertight. A less transient soft tissue finding associated with a previous anterior dislocation is a change in the size and, far more importantly, the configuration of the medial joint capsule (Figs. 7-2, 7-12). On the standing internal and external rotation views in normal individuals, there is an indentation between the axillary recess and subscapularis bursa, giving the medial capsule a figure "3" configuration (Fig. 7-9). In patients with a previous anterior dislocation, the indentation is lost, giving the medial capsule a smooth rounded contour [13] (Fig. 7-12). This arthrographic change can be attributed to the formation of an abnormal subperiosteal pocket of the glenoid created by the medial displacement of the humeral head [22]. This subperiosteal compartment persists, communicates with the capsule, and changes its appearance and contour. Although this arthrographic finding is a reliable sign of a previous anterior dislocation and is suggestive of an incompetent capsule, it is only observed in 15 percent of cases [7]. In addition to the leakage of contrast material and change in shape of the medial capsule, a third soft tissue sign is enlargement of the anterior capsule, as seen on the axillary or antero-posterior views. Enlargement of the axillary pouch [9], enlargement of the subscapularis bursa [13], and general enlargement [12] have all been observed. It has been the experience at the Hospital for Special Surgery that the size of the various portions of the anterior aspect of the joint capsule, like the nose on one's face, is extremely variable. Unless this qualitative finding is dramatic or accompanied by the altered configuration of the medial joint capsule, it is difficult to evaluate accurately.

The osteocartilaginous sequelae of an anterior dislocation can only be evaluated on double contrast arthrograms, which outline the articular cartilages of the joint (Fig. 7-13). These osteocartilaginous fractures are the result of the impact of the humeral head on the glenoid rim as it dislocates anteriorly (Fig. 7-14). The presence of cartilage injuries indicates that at least one dislocation has

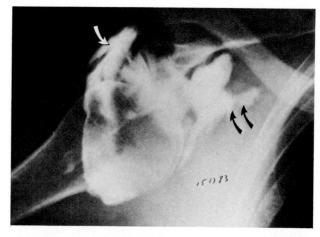

FIGURE 7-10. *Capsular leakage of contrast secondary to a subcoracoid anterior dislocation.*

The leakage (curved black arrows) is occurring from the superolateral and medial aspects of the capsule. The shoulder redislocated during the contrast study and the humeral head is out of the glenoid.

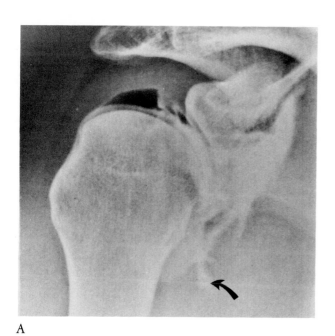

A

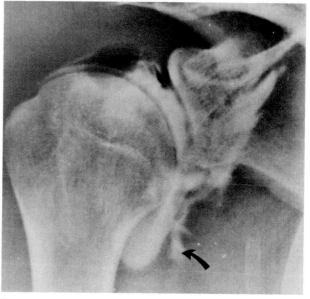

B

FIGURE 7-11. *Capsular extravasation of contrast material secondary to a recent subcoracoid anterior dislocation.*

A, B. The leakage has occurred from the inferomedial aspect of the capsule (curved black arrows), which would not occur simply from an excessive injection of contrast or from a contracted capsule.

Source: Courtesy of Dr. Jeremy Kaye.

114

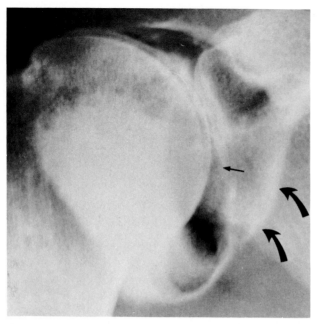

A

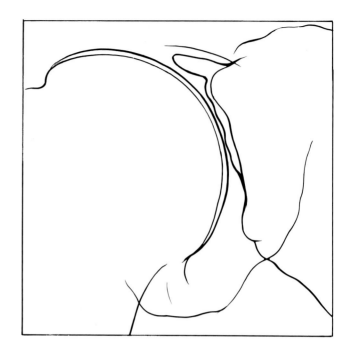

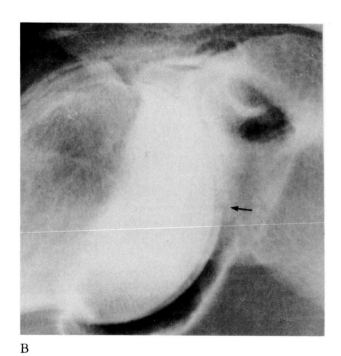

B

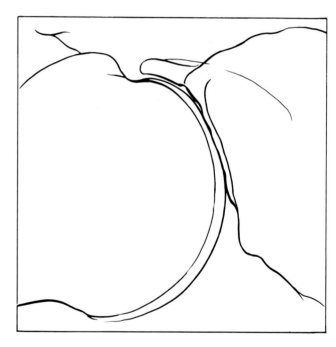

FIGURE 7-12. *Postdislocation changes in the medial margin of the capsule and a Bankart deformity.*

The routine standing external rotation view, A, reveals the medial capsule to be enlarged and smooth. There is loss of the normal indentation between the axillary recess and subscapularis bursa (curved black arrows). The routine standing external rotation view, A, and a second film with the arm elevated, B, demonstrate loss of the inferior glenoid labrum (black arrow).

Source: Goldman, A. B. Double Contrast Shoulder Arthrography. In R. H. Freiberger and J. J. Kaye (Eds.), *Arthrography.* New York: Appleton-Century-Crofts, 1979. P. 186.

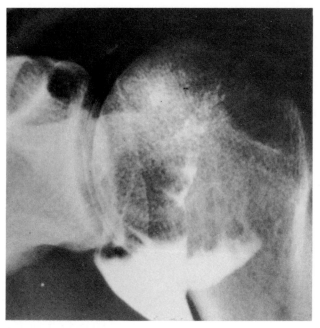

A

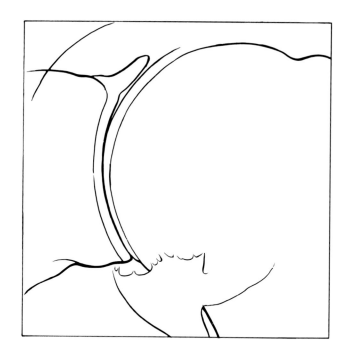

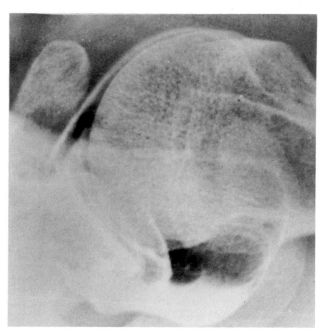

B

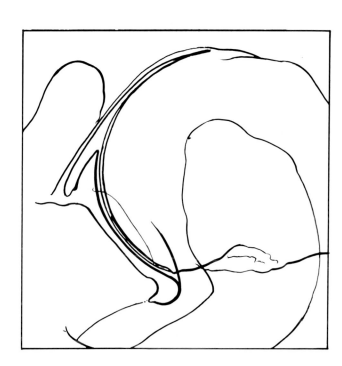

FIGURE 7-13. *Normal glenoid labrum.*
The glenoid as seen on the standing external rotation, A, and supine axillary, B, views. The cartilage of the glenoid is continuous, smooth, and concave. On the axillary view, B, the anterior labrum is triangular in shape and the posterior labrum is rounded.

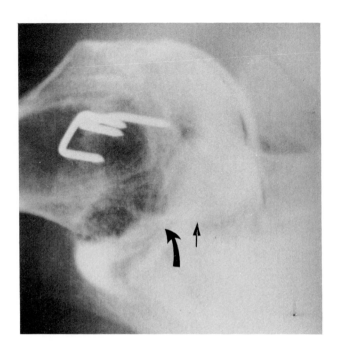

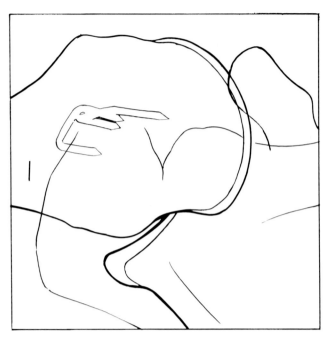

FIGURE 7-14. *Bankart and Hill-Sachs defects.*
An axillary view of double contrast arthrogram reveals the patient to have redislocated. The posterior cartilage of the humeral head (straight black arrow) is impacted against the anterior cartilage of the glenoid (curved black arrow), resulting in the Hill-Sachs and Bankart deformities.

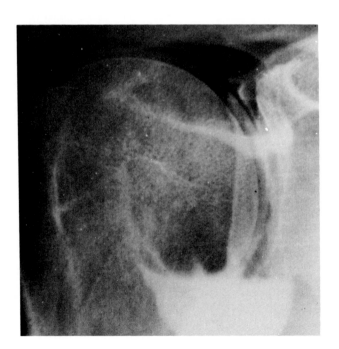

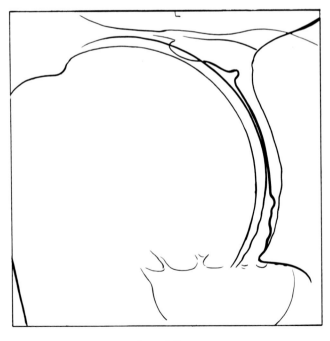

FIGURE 7-15. *Bankart defect.*
The standing external rotation view demonstrates irregularity and narrowing of the inferior aspect of the articular cartilage of the glenoid.

occurred. However, they do not reflect chronicity or repetitive dislocations. The Bankart defect [2], a compression or avulsion fracture of the anterior inferior glenoid labrum, has particular significance since it confirms the presence of an anterior dislocation, and its size and extent can indicate the direction of the dislocation. As on plain films, the term *Bankart defect* is now applied to the entire spectrum of post-traumatic osteocartilaginous deformities of the glenoid that follow an anterior dislocation. These injuries are usually limited to the fibrous labrum and/or articular cartilage and therefore are less frequently seen on plain films than the Hill-Sachs lesion. However, with the use of a double contrast technique, cartilage abnormalities can be demonstrated. The optimum routine views used in the evaluation of the glenoid rim are (1) the overpenetrated standing external rotation projection with the patient obliqued 25° posteriorly to view the joint in tangent and (2) the supine axillary view with most of the positive contrast material pooled posteriorly and the anterior glenoid labrum outlined by air.

On the external rotation view, the normal glenoid labrum is seen as a soft tissue density, which, on the arthrogram, is outlined by a thin smooth line of contrast material (Fig. 7-13). It is concave toward the humeral head and its superior and inferior borders are triangular in shape and wider than the midportion (Fig. 7-13). The Bankart deformity is identified on the arthrogram by the absence or irregularity of the anterior and/or inferior portion of the glenoid (Figs. 7-15, 7-16). If the entire width of the labrum has been avulsed, air and/or contrast outlines the subchondral bone (Fig. 7-17). If excessive contrast material has been injected and is pooling in the axillary pouch, it can obscure the base of the glenoid labrum. Repeat external rotation views can be obtained with

1. The arm elevated to stretch the capsule (Fig. 7-12)
2. The beam angled downward 25° to project the contrast in the axillary recess below the articular cartilage (Fig. 7-18A)
3. In the Trendelenburg position with the contrast pooled superiorly (Fig. 7-18B)

On the supine axillary view, the normal anterior glenoid labrum is triangular in shape with a sharp pointed superior tip (Fig. 7-13B). Following an

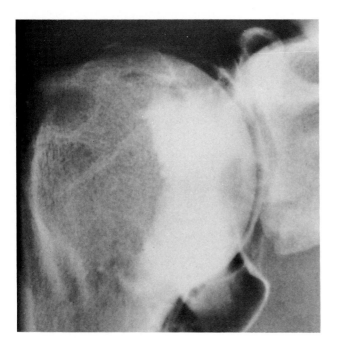

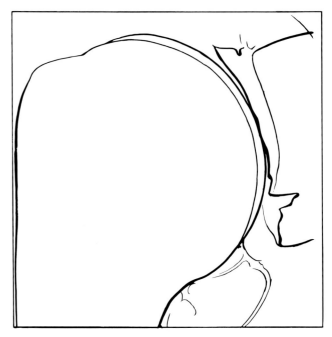

FIGURE 7-16. *Bankart defect.*
The external rotation view of a double contrast study shows complete avulsion of the articular cartilage of the inferior glenoid as well as an osseous compression fracture.

FIGURE 7-17. *Bankart defect.* ▶

A. The external rotation view shows air outlining the inferior osseous glenoid (black arrow) and an absence of articular cartilage.
B. The axillary view shows irregularity of the entire glenoid labrum suggesting that secondary degenerative joint disease has occurred after this patient's dislocation.

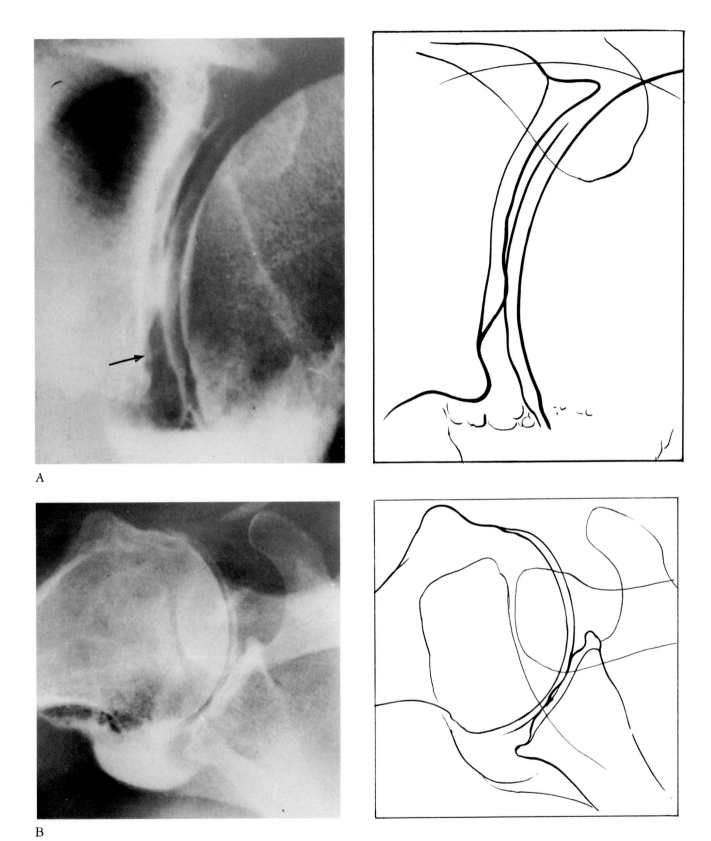

A

B

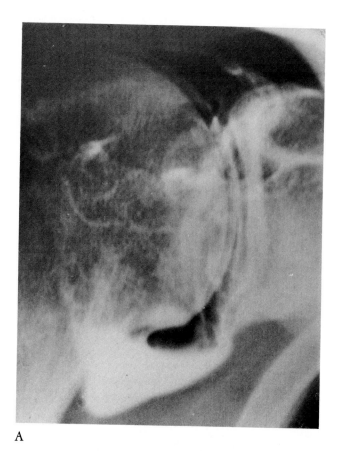

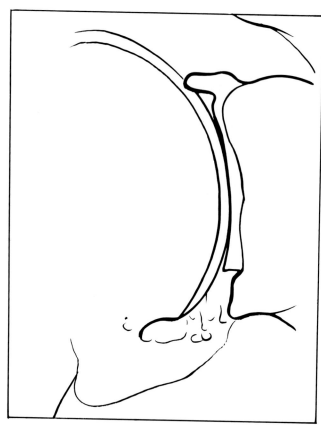

A

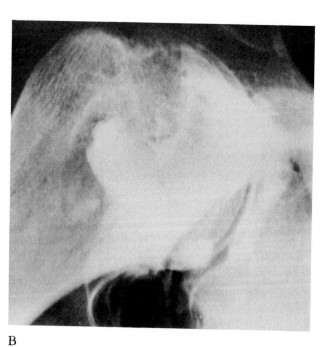

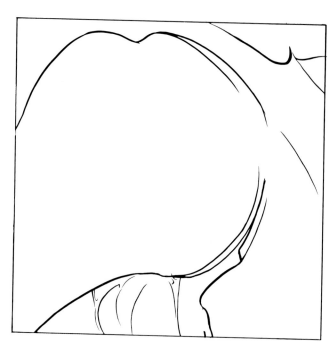

B

FIGURE 7-18. *Bankart defect.*
External rotation views were obtained with, A, the patient standing and beam angled 25° down toward the feet and, B, with the patient Trendelenburg and the arm elevated. Both views aid in visualizing the inferior glenoid labrum when too much positive contrast has been injected.

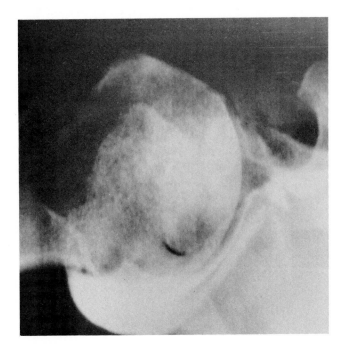

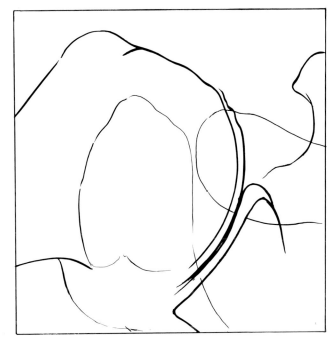

FIGURE 7-19. *Bankart defect.*
Supine axillary view shows abnormal rounding of anterior glenoid labrum.

anterior dislocation, blunting or amputation is frequently observed (Figs. 7-17, 7-19).

In most cases, routine views of the double contrast study determine the presence or absence of Bankart defects. However, the West Point prone axillary view, the Stryker view, and the Didiee view demonstrate various profiles of the humerus and glenoid (Fig. 7-20). Such additional studies can confirm equivocal cases, identify small defects not seen on the routine views, and further determine the direction of the injury. Occasionally, if the plain films are equivocal, tomograms may be of help (Figs. 7-21, 7-22). For tomography, the patient is placed supine on the table with the arm abducted 90° and the shoulder in external rotation (Figs. 7-21, 7-22). One-third centimeter linear tomographic cuts can then be obtained.

The Hill-Sachs compression defect is frequently seen on plain films but an occasional small or unusually placed defect can be identified solely on the basis of the double contrast study (Figs. 7-23 to 7-26).

Recognition of the presence and number of loose bodies is also important following a dislocation (Fig. 7-27). Twenty-five percent of patients with a previous anterior dislocation studied at the Hospital for Special Surgery with a double contrast technique, had one or more detached osteochondral fragments [6]. An extra set of internal and external rotation views, obtained with the patient supine can be helpful in distinguishing between true loose bodies and air bubbles.

Complete or partial rotator cuff tears are reported to occur in 10 percent of cases with an anterior dislocation [6] and can be demonstrated arthrographically (Figs. 7-24 to 7-26).

Posterior Dislocations, Posterior Subluxations, and Multidirectional Dislocators

The normal posterior glenoid labrum is a smooth, rounded structure (Fig. 7-28). Following a posterior dislocation, the prone axillary view of the arthrogram can demonstrate avulsion (Fig. 7-29) or "squaring" (Fig. 7-30). A cartilage compression defect on the medial aspect of the humeral head may also be present (Fig. 7-31). The arthrographic evaluation of a patient with a suspected posterior dislocation or subluxation should include the entire instability series since some of these patients dislocate in more than one direction.

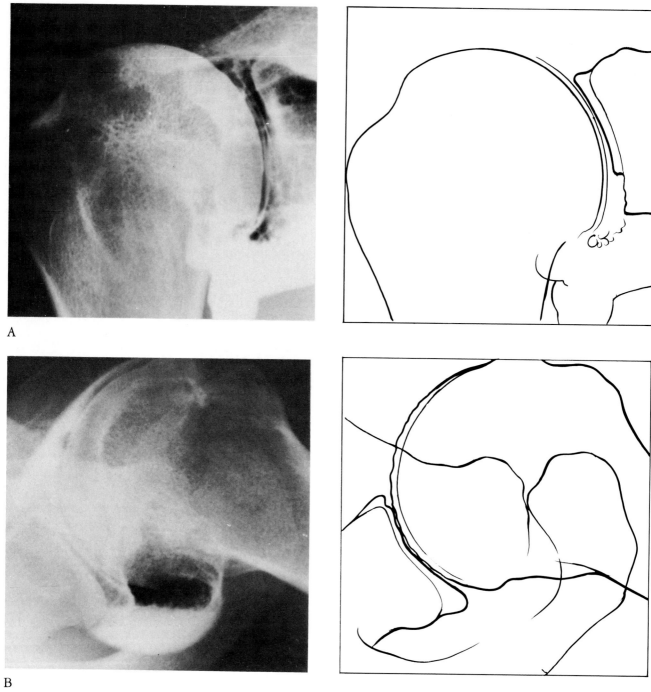

A

B

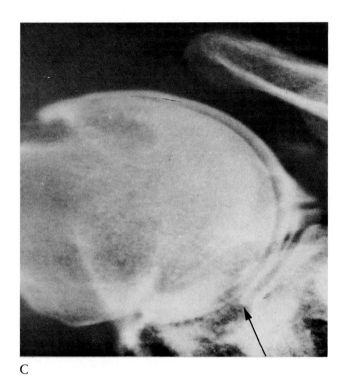

C

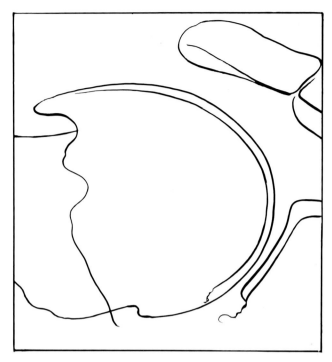

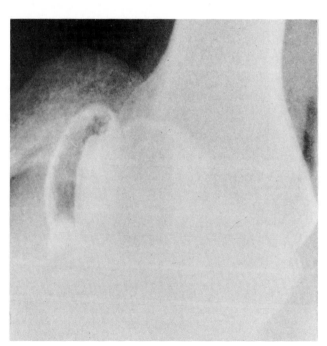

D

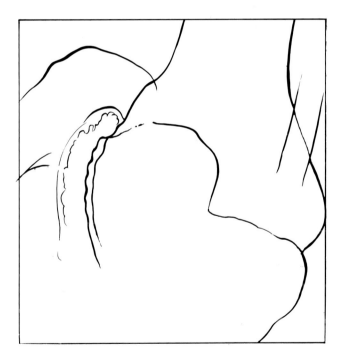

FIGURE 7-20.   *Cartilage Hill-Sachs and Bankart defects documented on the instability series.*

A. The standing external rotation view reveals irregularity of the inferior glenoid labrum.

B. The axillary view shows irregularity of both the anterior cartilage of the humeral head and the anterior glenoid labrum.

C. The Didiee view shows avulsion of the inferior glenoid labrum (black arrow).

D. The Stryker view reveals irregularity of the entire posterior articular surface of the humerus.

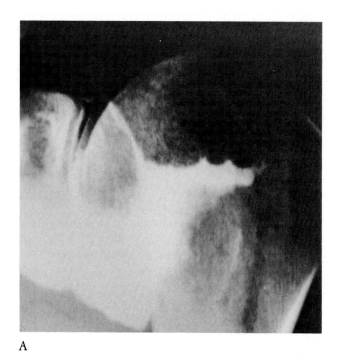

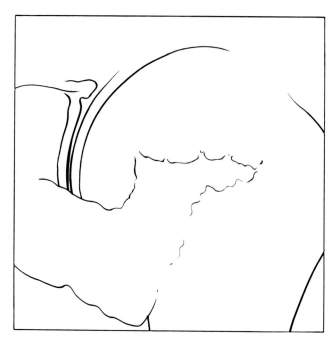

A

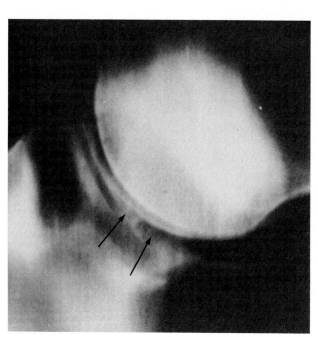

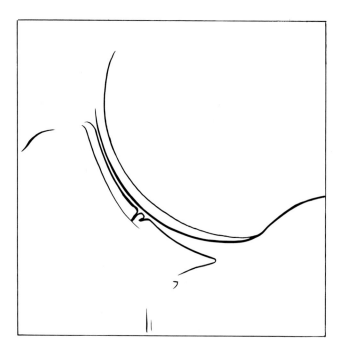

B

FIGURE 7-21. *Bankart defect.*

A. The standing external rotation view revealed excessive positive contrast material obscuring the inferior glenoid.

B. Tomograms obtained with the patient supine and the arm abducted 90° demonstrated the post-traumatic irregularity of the inferior half of the glenoid labrum (black arrows).

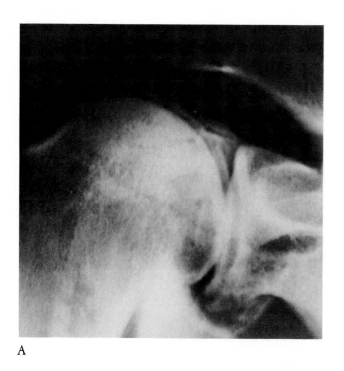
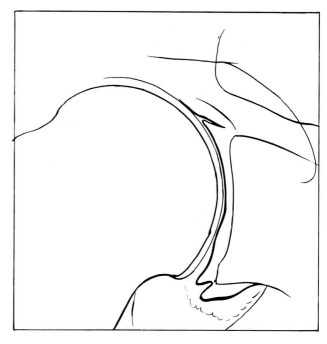

A

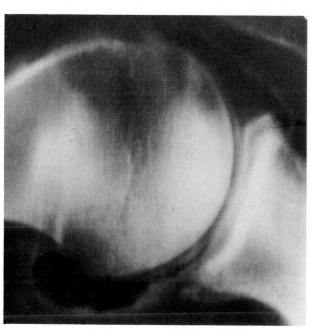
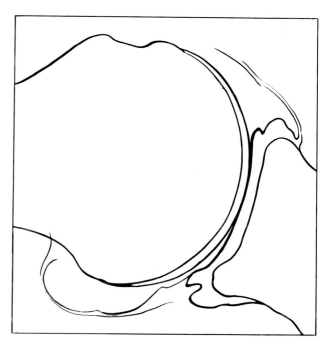

B

FIGURE 7-22. *Bankart deformity.*
Following an anterior dislocation, the inferior glenoid labrum has an abnormal "beak like" shape as seen on both the routine arthrogram films, A, and on a tomographic study, B.

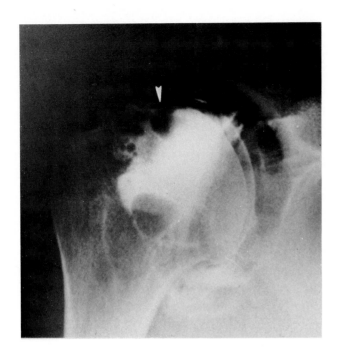

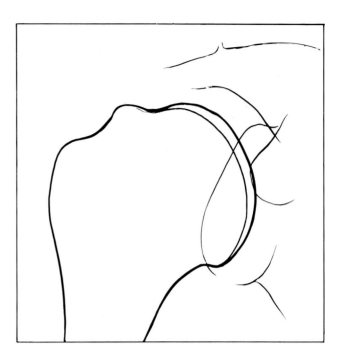

FIGURE 7-23. *Hill-Sachs deformity.*
This unusual superior cartilaginous compression defect on the humeral head (white arrowhead) suggests that the patient experienced a subglenoid anterior dislocation as opposed to the more common subcoracoid dislocation. A subcoracoid dislocation would have resulted in a more laterally placed compression fracture.

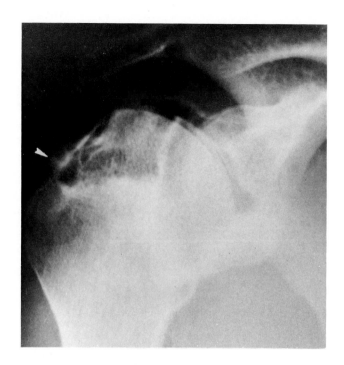 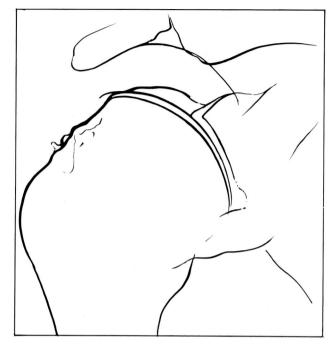

FIGURE 7-24.   *Hill-Sachs deformity and small partial rotator cuff tear (white arrowhead) shown on the standing internal rotation view.*

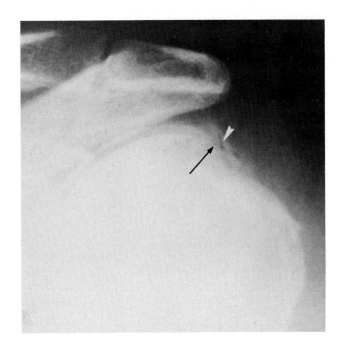
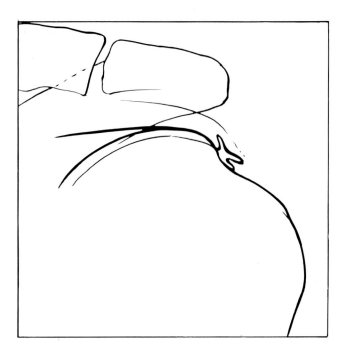

FIGURE 7-25. *Hill-Sachs deformity (black arrow) and partial rotator cuff tear (white arrowhead) demonstrated on a standing internal rotation view.*

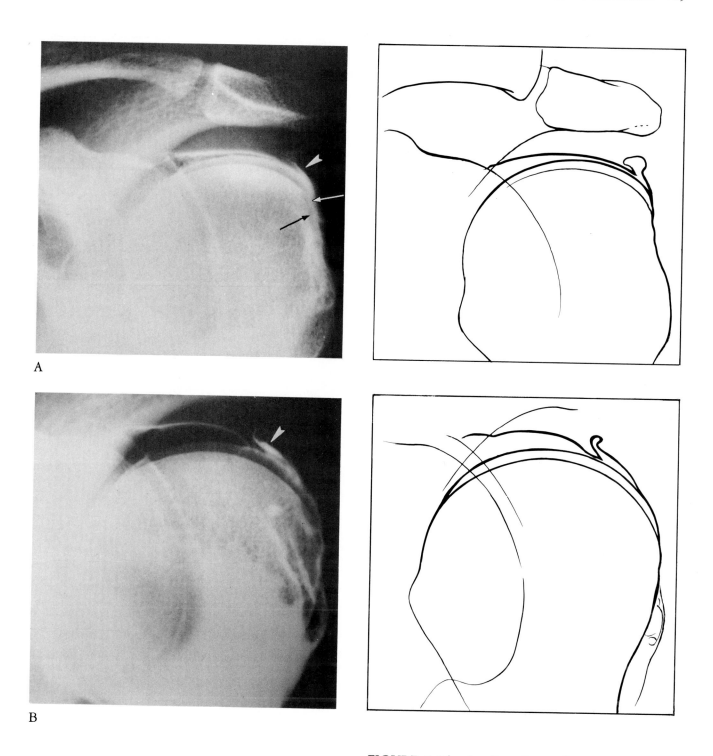

FIGURE 7-26. *Small cartilage Hill-Sachs deformity.*
Seen on only one standing internal rotation view (black arrow). Because of its small size a second study, B, with a slightly different degree of rotation failed to show the cartilage abnormality. Both internal rotation views reveal a partial rotator cuff tear (white arrowhead).

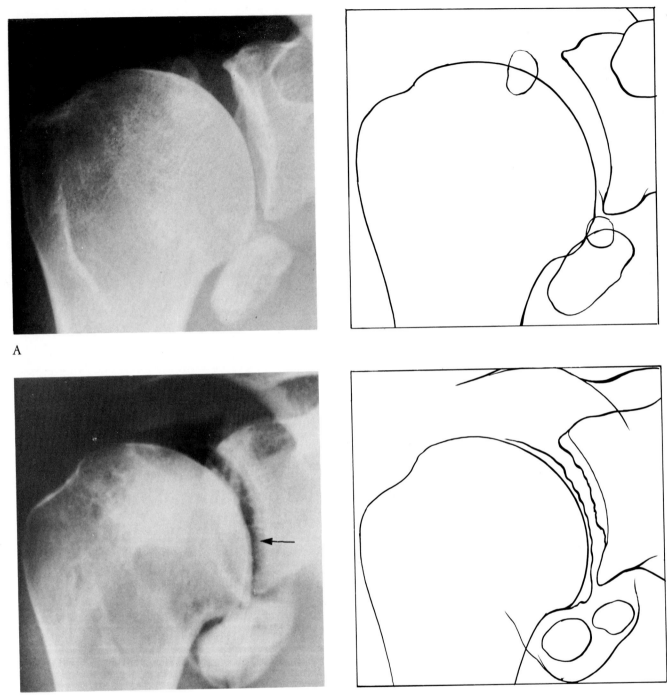

A

B

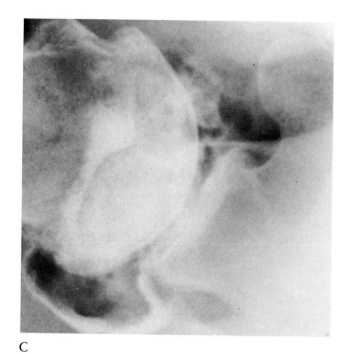

C

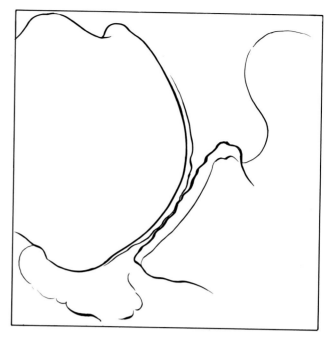

FIGURE 7-27. *Multiple loose bodies.*
Seen on the preliminary film, A, and on the standing external rotation view, B, and axillary view, C, of the arthrogram. The contrast study, B, also demonstrates a Bankart defect (black arrow) and a generalized narrowing and irregularity of the articular cartilages consistent with degenerative joint disease.

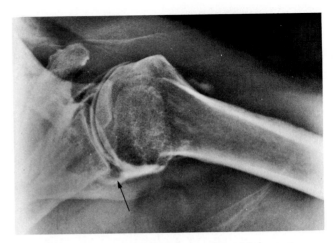

FIGURE 7-28. *Normal posterior glenoid labrum is smooth, rounded, and continuous with the concave articular surface of the glenoid (black arrow).*

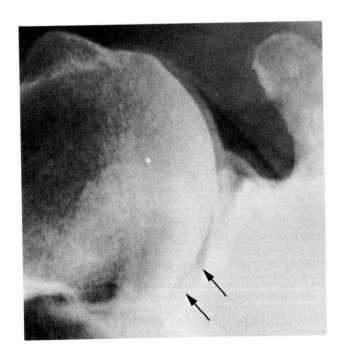

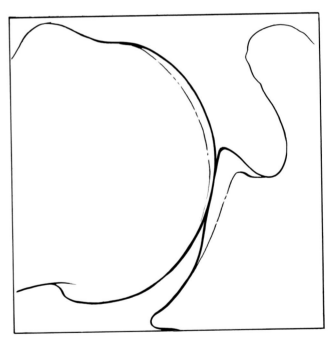

FIGURE 7-29. *Avulsion of the posterior glenoid labrum (black arrows) following a posterior dislocation of the humeral head, as demonstrated on the axillary view.*

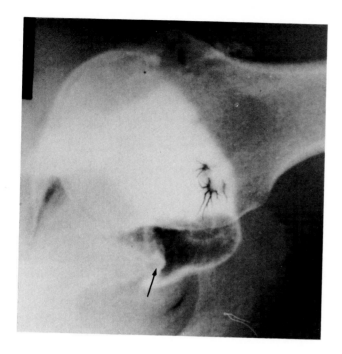

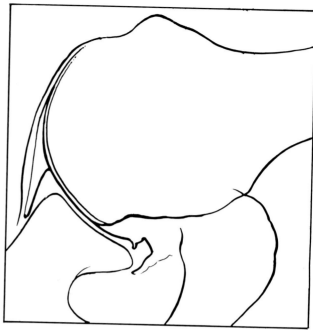

FIGURE 7-30. *Multidirectional dislocator.*
The prone axillary view reveals squaring of the posterior glenoid labrum, indicating a previous posterior dislocation (black arrow). The prone study also demonstrates anterior subluxation of the humeral head.

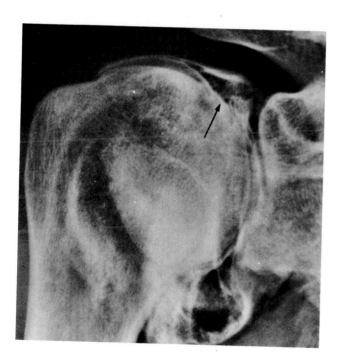

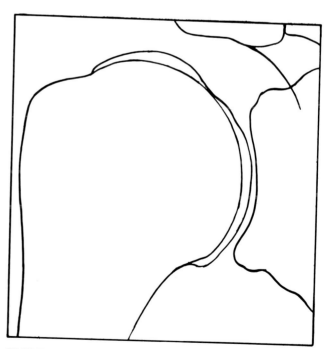

FIGURE 7-31. *Superomedial compression deformity of the cartilage of the humeral head (black arrow) secondary to a previous posterior dislocation of the humeral head.*
In this patient the so-called trough sign [5] was small and purely cartilaginous and seen only on the double contrast study.

CAUSES OF MISINTERPRETATION

False-negative studies are common and due primarily to technical difficulties: use of too much positive contrast material, failure to order the "instability series," failure to give epinephrine so that the edges of the articular cartilages become blurred, and contrast material injected subcutaneously.

False-positive studies occur if too much reliance is placed on the capsular findings of an anterior dislocation. Extravasation of contrast material due to a traumatic tear can be mimicked by extravasation from the normal weak points of the joint capsule (the subscapularis bursa and biceps tendon sheath), as a result of adhesive capsulitis, or finally as a result of a partial subcutaneous injection. Evaluation of the size of the capsule is a qualitative judgment, and unless the normal indentation between the axillary recess and subscapularis bursa is obliterated, it is far from reliable.

TREATMENT

Early reduction of an anterior glenohumeral dislocation is important as muscle spasm increases with time and reduction becomes progressively more difficult. There is also an increased incidence of neurovascular complications if treatment is delayed. A variety of methods are used for reduction. All depend on muscle relaxation and in certain cases even general anesthesia may be needed to achieve the necessary laxity. One of the simplest techniques of reduction is the Simpson method, in which the patient is placed prone on the table with the arm dangling over the side and a weight attached to the wrist. In some cases, spontaneous reduction occurs. In other cases, gentle traction on the arm while simultaneously putting pressure on the humeral head may achieve reduction. Recently, it has been noted that by rotating the scapula in a downward and outward plane, reduction occurs without forceful traction to the arm [3]. Another method of closed reduction is to hold the patient's wrist while slowly elevating the arm in a forward flexion plane. Spontaneous reduction usually occurs during this maneuver. More vigorous methods such as violent traction of the arm or the Kocher maneuver may result in neurovascular damage or fracture.

Surgery is usually reserved for patients who have recurrent dislocations or subluxations that interfere with sports or daily activities. Due to the many factors that predispose to recurrent injuries, several procedures are available. Surgical procedures to correct shoulder instability may be divided into four groups based on the anatomical approach: (1) tightening of the soft tissues about the shoulder and reattachment of the capsule to the glenoid to prevent instability, (2) bone blocks placed anteriorly or posteriorly to increase the width and depth of the glenoid cavity, (3) glenoid or humeral neck osteotomies that alter the forces controlling joint stability, and (4) tendon transfer procedures directed toward reinforcing joint stability [4]. All four types of procedures result in some loss of shoulder motion. At the Hospital for Special Surgery, the Bankart procedure (reattachment of the labrum and capsule to their anatomic position and tightening of the capsule) is considered the procedure of choice since loss of motion is minimized. Bone grafting procedures are reserved for those cases with Bankart defects affecting more than 40 percent of the glenoid surface.

Preoperative radiologic assessment of the shoulder can be important in determining the type of shoulder surgery indicated. The quality of the bone stock, particularly the glenoid margin, the presence of loose bodies, the size of the Hill-Sachs lesion, and the presence of rotator cuff tears should be studied. These parameters provide important information for the orthopaedic surgeon in preoperative planning.

REFERENCES

1. Adams, J. C. Recurrent dislocation of the shoulder. *J. Bone Joint Surg.* 30(B):26, 1948.
2. Bankart, A. S. B. The pathology and treatment of recurrent dislocation of the shoulder joint. *Br. J. Surg.* 26:23, 1938.
3. Bosley, R. C., and Miles, J. S. Scapula manipulation for reduction of anterior dislocation of the shoulder. Presented to the American Academy of Orthopedic Surgeons, San Francisco, California, 1979.
4. Boyd, H. B., and Hunt, M. D. Recurrent dislocation of the shoulder. The staple capsulorrhaphy. *J. Bone Joint Surg.* 47(A):1514, 1965.
5. Cisternino, S. J., Rogers, L. F., Bradley, C. S., et al. The trough line. A radiographic sign of posterior shoulder dislocation. *A.J.R.* 130:951, 1978.
6. El-Khoury, G. Y., Albright, J. P., Abu Yousef, M. M., et al. Arthrotomography of the glenoid labrum. *Radiology* 131:333, 1979.

7. Goldman, A. B., and Ghelman, B. The double contrast shoulder arthrogram. A review of 158 studies. *Radiology* 127:655, 1978.

8. Kinnett, J. G., Warren, R. F., and Jacobs, B. Recurrent dislocation of the shoulder after the age of 50. *Clin. Orthop.* 149:164, 1980.

9. Kummell, B. M. Arthrography of the anterior capsular derangement of the shoulder. *Clin. Orthop.* 83:170, 1972.

10. Moseley, H. F. *Shoulder Lesions* (3rd ed.). Edinburgh: Livingstone, 1969. Pp. 37–51.

11. Neer, C. S., II, and Foster, C. R. Inferior capsular shift for involuntary inferior and multidirectional instability of the shoulder. *J. Bone Joint Surg.* 62(A):897, 1980.

12. Nixon, J. R., and Young, W. S. Arthrography of the shoulder in anterior dislocation. A study of African and Asian patients. *Injury* 9:287, 1978.

13. Reeves, B. Arthrography of the shoulder. Anterior dislocations. *J. Bone Joint Surg.* 48(B):424, 1966.

14. Reeves, B. Experiments on the tensile strength of the anterior capsular structures of the shoulder in man. *J. Bone Joint Surg.* 50(B):858, 1968.

15. Rokous, J. R., Feagin, J. A., and Abbott, H. G. Modified axillary roentgenograms. A useful adjunct in the diagnosis of recurrent instability of the shoulder. *Clin. Orthop.* 82:84, 1972.

16. Rowe, C. R. Symposium on surgical lesions of the shoulder. Acute and recurrent dislocations of the shoulder. *J. Bone Joint Surg.* 44(A):977, 1962.

17. Rowe, C. R. Anterior dislocations of the shoulder. *Surg. Clin. North Am.* 43:1609, 1963.

18. Rowe, C. R., Patel, D., and Southmayd, W. W. The Bankart procedure. A long-term end result study. *J. Bone Joint Surg.* 60(A):1, 1978.

19. Rowe, C. R. Anterior dislocation of the shoulder. *Orthop. Clin. North Am.* 11:253, 1980.

20. Rubin, S. A., Gray, R. L., and Green, W. B. Scapula "Y" view. A diagnostic aid in shoulder trauma. *Radiology* 110:725, 1974.

21. Symeonides, P. P. The significance of the subscapularis muscle in the pathogenesis of recurrent anterior dislocations of the shoulder. *J. Bone Joint Surg.* 54(B):476, 1972.

22. Tijmes, J., Loyd, J. M., and Tullos, H. S. Arthrography in acute shoulder dislocations. *South. Med. J.* 72:564, 1979.

23. Turkel, S. J., Panio, M. W., Marshall, J. L., Girgis, F. G. Stabilizing mechanism preventing anterior dislocation of the glenohumeral joint. *J. Bone Joint Surg.* 63(A):1208, 1981.

SUGGESTED READING

Aston, J. W., and Gregory, C. F. Dislocation of the shoulder with significant fracture of the glenoid. *J. Bone Joint Surg.* 55(A):1531, 1973.

Bateman, J. E. *The Shoulder and Neck* (2nd ed.). Philadelphia: Saunders, 1978. Pp. 490–519.

Bost, F. C., and Imman, V. T. The pathological changes

in recurrent dislocation of the shoulder. A report of Bankart's operative procedure. *J. Bone Joint Surg.* 24(A):595, 1942.

Boyd, H. B., and Sish, T. D. Recurrent posterior dislocation of the shoulder. *J. Bone Joint Surg.* 54(A):779, 1972.

Braunstein, E. M., and Martel, W. Voluntary glenohumeral dislocation. *A. J. R.* 129:911, 1977.

Bush, L. E. The torn shoulder capsule. *J. Bone Joint Surg.* 57(A):256, 1975.

Collins, H. R., and Wilde, A. H. Shoulder instability in athletes. *Orthop. Clin. North Am.* 4:759, 1973.

DePalma, A. F. *Surgery of the Shoulder* (2nd ed.). Philadelphia: Lippincott, 1973. Pp. 403–425.

DePalma, A. F., and Flannery, G. F. Acute anterior dislocation of the shoulder. *J. Sports Med.* 1:6, 1973.

Dutoit, G. T., and Roux, D. Recurrent dislocations of shoulder. Twenty-four year study of the Johannesburg stapling operation. *J. Bone Joint Surg.* 37(A):633, 1955.

Kerwein, G. A., Roseberg, B., and Sneed, W. R., Jr. Arthrographic studies of the shoulder joint. *J. Bone Joint Surg.* 39(A):1267, 1957.

Kessel, L. Injuries of the Shoulder. In J. N. Wilson (ed.), *Watson-Jones Fractures and Joint Injuries* (5th ed.). Edinburgh and London: Churchill Livingstone, 1976. Pp. 521–586.

Killoran, P. J., Marcove, R. C., and Freiberger, R. H. Shoulder arthrography. *A. J. R.* 103:658, 1968.

Magnuson, P. B. Treatment of recurrent dislocation of the shoulder. *Surg. Clin. North Am.* 25:14, 1945.

May, V. R., Jr. A modified Bristow operation for anterior recurrent dislocation of the shoulder. *J. Bone Joint Surg.* 52(A):1010, 1970.

May, V. R., Jr. Posterior dislocation of the shoulder. *Orthop. Clin. North Am.* 11:271, 1980.

McLaughlin, M. L. Posterior dislocation of the shoulder. *J. Bone Joint Surg.* 44(A):1477, 1962.

Mink, J. H., Richardson, A., and Grant, T. T. Evaluation of glenoid labrum by double contrast shoulder arthrography. *A. J. R.* 133:883, 1979.

Neer, C. S., II, and Welsh, R. P. The shoulder in sports. *Orthop. Clin. North Am.* 8:583, 1977.

Nelson, D. H. Arthrography of the shoulder joint. *Br. J. Radiol.* 25:134, 1952.

Neviaser, J. S. Posterior dislocation of the shoulder. Diagnosis and treatment. *Surg. Clin. North Am.* 43:1623, 1963.

Pavlov, H., and Freiberger, R. H. Fractures and dislocations about the shoulder. *Semin. Roentgenol.* 13:85, 1978.

Preston, B. J., and Jackson, J. P. Investigation of shoulder disability by arthrography. *Clin. Radiol.* 28:259, 1977.

Rockwood, C. A., and Green, D. P. *Fractures.* Philadelphia: Lippincott, 1975. Pp. 624–718.

Samilson, R. L., Raphael, R. L., Post, L., et al. Shoulder arthrography. *J.A.M.A.* 175:773, 1961.

Scott, D. J., Jr. Treatment of recurrent posterior dislocations of the shoulder by glenoplasty. Report of three cases. *J. Bone Joint Surg.* 49(A):471, 1967.

8

Capsular Deformities: Adhesive Capsulitis

The terms *frozen shoulder* and *adhesive capsulitis* refer to a clinical syndrome characterized by a painful decrease of glenohumeral motion. The etiology, pathology, and treatment remain controversial. In many instances, prolonged disuse is the precipitating factor. The cause of the disuse may be an abnormality of the osseous structures, the articular cartilages, or the surrounding ligaments. Trauma or inflammation of any of these structures can result in muscle spasm and immobilization. Much of the confusion surrounding adhesive capsulitis results from the difficulty in separating the changes produced by the presence of two coexisting abnormalities. As stated by DePalma, "this is like trying to decipher the riddle of the chicken and the egg—which came first" [5].

ANATOMY REVIEW

The shoulder joint is a tightly enclosed structure in which the capsule of the glenohumeral joint lies in close approximation to the rotator cuff, the subacromial bursa, the coracoacromial ligament, and the acromion process. Therefore, any lesion involving these structures, such as the impingement syndrome with rotator cuff inflammation, calcific peritendinitis, or biceps tendinitis, may produce anterior shoulder pain and initiate the frozen shoulder syndrome [7].

The synovial-lined joint capsule normally inserts on the humeral head just proximal to the greater tuberosity, crosses medially at the level of the anatomic neck of the humerus, and attaches to the osseous rim of the glenoid (Fig. 8-1). The axillary recess is an area of redundancy that hangs between the humerus and scapula and permits elevation of the arm (Fig. 8-1). Surrounding the capsule and incorporated into it is the thick, tendinous rotator cuff. It, in turn, is encased by the subacromial-subdeltoid bursa. The osseous acromioclavicular arch and the coracoacromial ligament surround and fix the soft tissue integuments of the shoulder. The tendon of the long head of the biceps lies within the joint capsule from its origin to the bicipital groove, and at the level of the groove it is in intimate contact with the capsule and supraspinatus tendon.

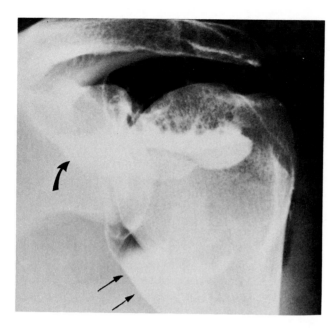

FIGURE 8-1. *Normal capsule.*
An external rotation view shows the insertion along the humeral neck, the axillary recess (black arrows), and the subscapularis bursa (black curved arrow). Note that the capsular insertion has a smooth contour.

PATHOPHYSIOLOGY

The etiology of the frozen shoulder syndrome is controversial. Bateman [3] and Neviaser [9, 10, 11] have reported series of patients with primary idiopathic adhesive capsulitis and no predisposing factors (Figs. 8-2 to 8-5). However, in other series, most cases are initiated by and secondary to prolonged disuse. The precipitating factor may be within the shoulder (bicipital tendinitis, calcific peritendinitis, rotator cuff inflammation, fractures; Figs. 8-6 to 8-9) or from extra-articular abnormalities (angina pectoris, cervical spondylosis). The incidence of these preexisting conditions is also in doubt. Various investigators have incriminated bicipital tendinitis [5], acromioclavicular abnormalities [3], or tendinitis of the rotator cuff [9, 10, 11] as the most frequent primary abnormalities. Again, the apparent confusion results from the difficulty in distinguishing primary changes from secondary changes and deciding if the capsular abnormalities resulted in the inflammation of the surrounding structures or vice versa.

Although most researchers agree that immobility is the most important factor in the etiology of the frozen shoulder, Bateman has pointed out that since the syndrome does not occur in quadriplegics, there must be other variables [3]. Among other predisposing conditions is, first, the age of the patient. Adhesive capsulitis does not occur in young individuals but is common in middle age. Second, reflex muscle spasm is important in initiating the fibrotic changes.

Regardless of the initiating cause of the frozen shoulder, the pathology is the same. The frozen shoulder is characterized by thickening of the entire joint capsule by fibrous tissue that is compact and cellular [8]. Due to the formation of intraarticular adhesions, the synovial lining becomes adherent to the adjacent articular cartilage [8]. Synovial fluid is decreased or absent. All the surrounding soft tissues, particularly the supraspinatus tendon, are involved by similar pathologic changes [8]. The fibrotic coracohumeral ligament prevents normal external rotation. The normal sliding mechanism of the tendon of the long head of the biceps is also disrupted. Involvement of the biceps tendon contributes significantly to the anterior distribution of shoulder pain associated with adhesive capsulitis.

Inflammatory changes in the adjacent soft tissue structures have also been reported [4, 5]. It is

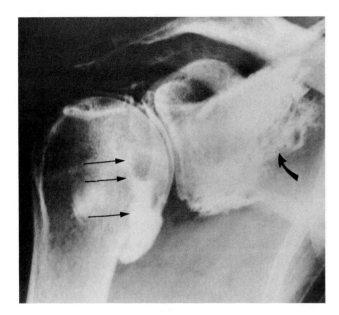

FIGURE 8-2.   *Primary adhesive capsulitis.*
The capsule is retracted away from the tuberosities (black arrows). The axillary recess is small, and extravasation has occurred prior to exercise (curved black arrow).

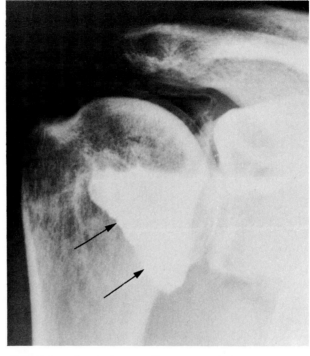

FIGURE 8-4.   *Primary adhesive capsulitis.*
The capsular margin is scalloped (black arrows), and the axillary recess is small.

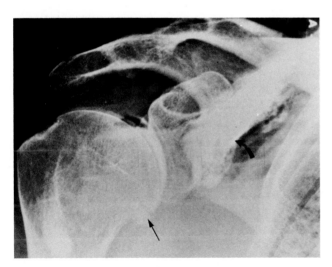

FIGURE 8-3.   *Primary adhesive capsulitis.*
This view shows almost complete extravasation of contrast through the subscapularis bursa (curved black arrow) and a tiny axillary recess (black arrow).

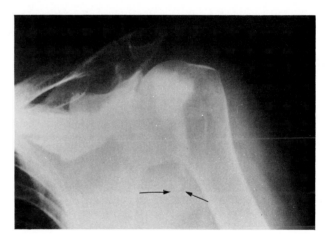

FIGURE 8-5.   *Primary adhesive capsulitis on single contrast study.*
The external rotation view shows a pinched-off pocket of contrast in the axilla (black arrows).

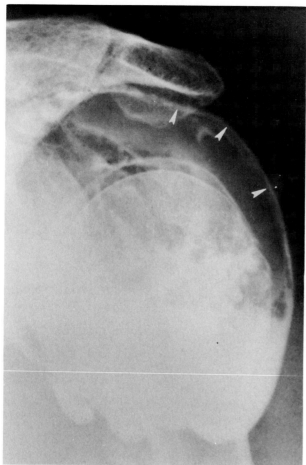

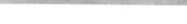

A

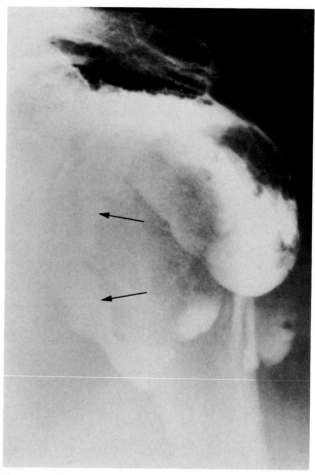

B

FIGURE 8-6. *Secondary adhesive capsulitis.*

A. The internal rotation view demonstrates a complete rotator cuff tear with contrast in the subacromial-subdeltoid bursa (white arrowheads).

B. The external rotation view demonstrates the capsular margin to be scalloped and retracted medially (black arrows).

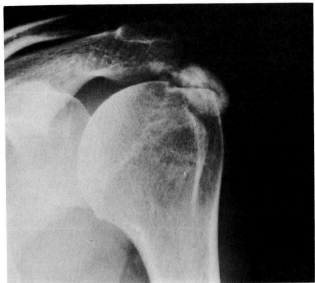

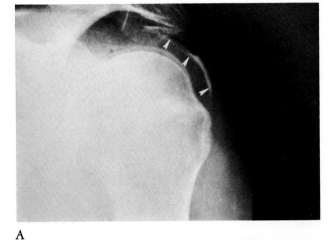

A

A

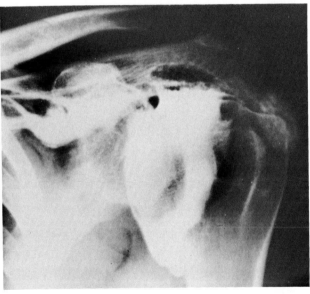

B

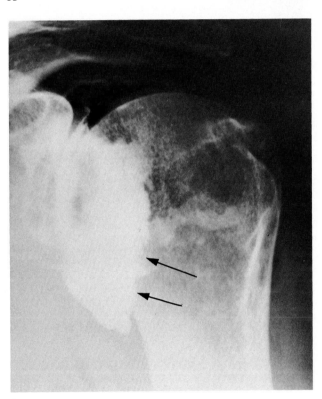

B

FIGURE 8-7.   *Secondary adhesive capsulitis.*
A. The plain film shows calcium in the region of the supraspinatus tendon.
B. The arthrogram reveals a small axillary recess and extravasation of contrast from the subscapularis bursa on the pre-exercise study.

FIGURE 8-8.   *Secondary adhesive capsulitis.*
A. The internal rotation view shows a complete rotator cuff tear with air and contrast within the subacromial-subdeltoid bursa (white arrowheads).
B. The external rotation view demonstrates retraction of the capsule away from the tuberosities, scalloping of the capsular margin (black arrows), and a small axillary recess.

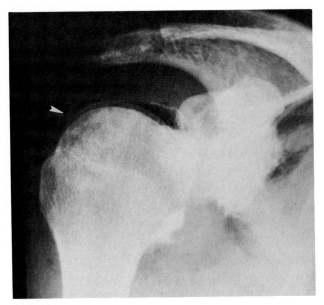

A

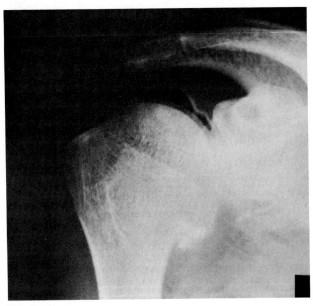

B

FIGURE 8-9. *Secondary adhesive capsulitis.*
The internal rotation view, A, shows a partial rotator cuff tear with air and contrast above the cartilage of the humeral head (white arrowhead). Both internal, A, and external, B, rotation views show extreme extravasation of contrast and no axillary recess at all.

uncertain whether the inflammation initiates the frozen shoulder syndrome, or whether the frozen shoulder syndrome produces the inflammatory reaction.

CLINICAL

The frozen shoulder syndrome occurs almost exclusively in the middle-aged individual. It affects females more frequently than males, and it preferentially involves the left shoulder. These observations have been attributed to the decreased physical activity in middle-aged females as opposed to males of the same age and the decreased use of the nondominant arm.

The presenting complaint of a patient with the frozen shoulder syndrome is usually pain initiated by minor trauma. The onset of symptoms is insidious, and pain is most intense along the anterior aspect of the shoulder and may be referred down the arm. As the pain increases in intensity, protective muscle spasm, primarily of the rotator cuff, deltoid, and pectoralis major ensues. The muscle spasm, in turn, results in a vicious cycle with further diminution of shoulder motion and further disuse.

The physical examination reveals limitation of motion as well as pain with motion. Abduction and rotation are severely limited. The anterior aspect of the shoulder and the course of the biceps tendon may be tender to palpation. Atrophy of the surrounding muscles is common.

The clinical course of patients with adhesive capsulitis is variable. Some improve spontaneously and regain most of the lost motion; others improve, but never achieve a normal range of motion, while still others remain severely disabled.

PLAIN FILMS

Plain film findings may be absent or there can be juxta-articular osteoporosis related to disuse. In cases with secondary adhesive capsulitis the findings vary and may include calcification in the region of the rotator cuff (Fig. 8-7), calcification in the tendon of the long head of the biceps, and loss of the normal space between the humeral head and acromion process indicating advanced degeneration of the rotator cuff. In general, the plain films are only suggestive and not diagnostic of adhesive capsulitis.

ARTHROGRAPHIC ABNORMALITIES

The shoulder arthrogram is performed for two reasons in patients who are clinically suspected of having the frozen shoulder syndrome. First, the contrast study can provide objective evidence of the capsular changes and, second, it can in some cases identify the primary underlying abnormality, such as trauma to the long head of the biceps or a tear of the rotator cuff that may require treatment. De-Palma emphasizes that in cases where the frozen shoulder syndrome is secondary to other pathology, the primary disorder must be eradicated before the capsular changes can be successfully addressed [5].

The arthrographic criteria for a frozen shoulder include

1. Pain following the injection of less than 10 cc of contrast material
2. Retraction of the joint capsule away from the greater tuberosity (Figs. 8-2 to 8-9)
3. Irregularity and scalloping of the capsular insertion (Figs. 8-4, 8-6)
4. A small axillary recess (Figs. 8-2 to 8-9), which may become "pinched-off" in external rotation (Fig. 8-5)
5. Extravasation of contrast material without injection of more than 10 cc of contrast material or exercise (Figs. 8-2 to 8-3)

At least two of these findings should be present to establish the diagnosis, since none are pathognomonic.

The first arthrographic sign that suggests the presence of adhesive capsulitis is the pain produced by the injection of contrast into the contracted joint capsule. The discomfort is probably caused by the forceful distention of the fibrosed inflamed capsule. Shoulder pain during the injection is most intense when the single contrast technique is employed. Air, when injected into a frozen shoulder, tends to leak rapidly into the interstitium, relieving the pressure and minimizing the pain produced by the injection. However, pain during a shoulder arthrogram may not arise from adhesive capsulitis but from technical difficulties.

The second and third roentgen criteria are medial retraction of the capsule away from the tuberosities and scalloping of the capsular margin. The scalloping of the capsular insertion is probably related to a combination of fibrotic and inflammatory changes. However, as an isolated finding, scalloping is not reliable. In the experience at the Hospital for Special Surgery many cases with scalloping have been observed with normal volume and no clinical evidence of a decreased range of motion. The reason for irregularity of the capsular margin in asymptomatic patients has never been determined.

The fourth diagnostic criterion is a small axillary recess. The axillary recess provides the normal redundancy that permits elevation of the arm. Therefore, the arthrographic demonstration of a small recess is visual evidence of loss of external rotation and abduction. In some cases, when the arm is externally rotated, the axillary recess becomes a small, rounded pocket that is apparently separated from the rest of the capsule. Although size alone is a qualitative judgment, a small axillary recess with a pinched-off appearance is the most reliable of the arthrographic criteria.

Extravasation of contrast material from the subscapularis bursa and biceps tendon sheath also should be carefully evaluated. The leakage of contrast from these two normally weak points in the joint capsule is related to mechanical factors: the volume of the capsule, the volume of the contrast injected, and the amount of intra-articular pressure generated by exercise. Unless the extravasation occurs prior to exercise and with the injection of only small amounts of contrast, it cannot be considered evidence of a frozen shoulder.

The second reason for performing the contrast study is to identify cases of secondary adhesive capsulitis. In cases with complete or partial tears of the rotator cuff, the etiology of the frozen shoulder is evident. However, in patients with abnormalities of the tendon of the long head of the biceps, the sequence of events is far from clear. Investigators disagree as to whether biceps tendinitis is the etiology of, or results from, the capsular abnormalities or whether both situations can occur.

In patients where adhesive capsulitis has already been diagnosed, shoulder arthrography can also be performed to attempt lysis of adhesions by repetitive, forceful distention of the joint capsule [1, 2, 6]. This technique is discussed below in the section on treatment.

CAUSES FOR MISINTERPRETATION OF THE ARTHROGRAM

Significant pain during the injection of contrast material can be the result of problems other than adhesive capsulitis. Active synovitis or recent trauma to the capsule can produce significant discomfort. Severe pain can also be associated with a partial interosseous injection when the needle is embedded between the cartilage and the bone. Such an injection produces a density in the humerus that resembles a medullary infarct. If the patient experiences pain during the injection of contrast, it is advisable to check the fluoroscopic image to rule out an interosseous injection.

False-negative interpretations in patients with adhesive capsulitis result from extensive extravasation of contrast material before films can be obtained. In cases of severe frozen shoulder, all of the air and contrast can leak out of the shoulder within a matter of minutes, and pathology in the rotator cuff or biceps tendon cannot be absolutely excluded. In such patients, it may be advisable to use a single contrast technique, although this technique does not always prevent leakage.

Failure to fill the biceps tendon sheath also limits the diagnostic significance of the study. As failure to fill may be due to pathology of either the capsule or the tendon, no conclusion can be drawn. With the single contrast technique, failure to fill the tendon sheath may also occur in normal individuals.

False-positive studies are usually the result of relying on a single criterion. Capsular irregularity has been observed in asymptomatic individuals. Extravasation of contrast can result from adhesive capsulitis, but it can also result from excessive injections of more than 12 cc of contrast. The size of the axillary recess is variable and unless it is very small, or pinched-off in its appearance, it is not an accurate criterion, since individual variations can be misinterpreted as pathology. It cannot be sufficiently emphasized that at least two arthrographic criteria should be present to reliably establish the diagnosis of a frozen shoulder.

TREATMENT

For cases of adhesive capsulitis that are secondary to intrinsic shoulder pathology or referred shoulder pain, treatment should be directed toward ameliorating the primary condition [5]. In patients with impingement syndrome, subacromial injections of local anesthesia or even acromioplasty may be required [7]. In patients with cervical spondylosis, neck immobilization should be combined with anti-inflammatory medications and cervical spine exercise.

In all patients with adhesive capsulitis regardless of etiology, initial treatment of the shoulder is directed toward achieving improvements in motion and encouraging the use of the shoulder in daily activity. In patients with markedly restricted motion (less than 90° of forward flexion), surgical and/or arthrographic brisement may be helpful [1, 2, 6]. During this procedure the joint is forcefully distended with lidocaine, saline and/or contrast material in an effort to disrupt local adhesions. The results of arthrographic brisement at the Hospital for Special Surgery have not been consistent. In many cases, it resulted in several hours of pain relief due to the large amounts of lidocaine administered during the procedure, but the relief was rarely sustained. A mild increase in range of motion (10°–20°) can be achieved, and if combined with an intensive program of physiotherapy, may result in some sustained improvement [6]. The more severe the adhesive capsulitis, the less likely this procedure is to help the patient.

In a small group of patients with advanced disease, surgical manipulation may be required. This procedure carries with it the dangers of tuberosity fractures and rotator cuff tears. Improved external rotation can be achieved but will only be sustained if followed by an intensive program of exercise.

REFERENCES

1. Andren, L., and Lundberg, B. J. Treatment of rigid shoulders by joint distention during arthrography. *Acta Orthop. Scand.* 36:45, 1965.
2. Annexton, M. Arthrography can help free "frozen shoulder." *J.A.M.A.* 241:875, 1979.
3. Bateman, A. S. B. *The Shoulder and Neck* (2nd ed.). Philadelphia: Saunders, 1978. Pp. 169, 367–370.
4. DePalma, A. F. The frozen shoulder. American Academy of Orthopedic Surgeons. Instructional Course Lecture IX:313–325, 1952.
5. DePalma, A. F. *Surgery of the Shoulder* (2nd ed.). Philadelphia: Lippincott, 1973. Pp. 450–468.
6. Gilula, L. A., Schoenecker, P. L., and Murphy, W. A. Shoulder arthrography as a treatment modality. *A. J. R.* 131:1047, 1978.
7. Killoran, P. J., Marcove, R. C., and Freiberger, R. H. Shoulder arthrography. *A.J.R.* 103:658, 1968.

8. Neer, C. S., II. Anterior acromioplasty for the chronic impingement syndrome in the shoulder. A preliminary report. *J. Bone Joint Surg.* 54(A):41, 1972.

9. Lundberg, B. J. The frozen shoulder. Clinical and radiographical observations. The effect of manipulation under general anesthesia. Structure and glycosaminoglycan content of the joint capsule. Local bone metabolism. *Acta Orthop. Scand.* (Suppl.) 119:1, 1969.

10. Neviaser, J. S. Adhesive capsulitis of the shoulder. A study of pathological findings in periarthritis of the shoulder. *J. Bone Joint Surg.* 27:211, 1945.

11. Neviaser, J. S. Adhesive capsulitis of the shoulder. *Am. Acad. Orthop. Surg.* Instructional Course Lectures. 6:281–291, 1949.

SUGGESTED READING

Codman, E. A. *The Shoulder.* New York: Miller, 1934. Pp. 118–119.

Grey, R. G. Natural history of "idiopathic frozen shoulder." *J. Bone Joint Surg.* 60(A):564, 1978.

Neviaser, J. S. Arthrography of the shoulder joint. Study of findings in adhesive capsulitis of the shoulder. *J. Bone Joint Surg.* 44(A):1321, 1962.

Neviaser, J. S. *Arthrography of the Shoulder. The Diagnosis and Management of the Lesion Visualized.* Springfield, Ill.: Thomas, 1975. Pp. 33–68.

Sisk, T. D., and Canale, S. T. Traumatic affections of joints. In A. M. Crenshaw (Ed.), Campbell's Operative Orthopaedics (5th ed.). St. Louis: Mosby, 1971. Pp. 1005–1006.

Samilson, R. L., Raphael, R. L., Post, L., et al. Shoulder arthrography. *J.A.M.A.* 175:773, 1961.

Other Abnormalities: Arthritides, Loose Bodies, Osteonecrosis, and Total Shoulder Replacement

CARTILAGE ABNORMALITIES
Arthritis

In the evaluation of arthritic changes, the shoulder arthrogram can be of help in several ways. First, the aspirated fluid may establish the diagnosis if it contains bacteria (septic arthritis) or blood in the absence of trauma (pigmented villonodular synovitis). Due to the depth of the shoulder joint, it is often difficult to obtain synovial fluid, and in cases of suspected arthritis, 10 milliliters of sterile saline, without bacteriocidal agents, should be injected and reaspirated. The saline can often displace synovial fluid that has dropped to the back of the shoulder joint. Second, the contrast study may demonstrate the intra-articular synovial masses that are characteristic of certain proliferative arthritides, such as pigmented villonodular synovitis, uncalcified synovial chondromatosis, and tuberculosis (Fig. 9-1). All three diseases have extensive synovial hypertrophy in the absence of obvious joint-space narrowing. Although the arthrogram can demonstrate the synovial abnormality, it cannot distinguish among these three diseases. Third, in patients with known arthritis, the arthrogram can demonstrate the severity of cartilage destruction and synovitis (Figs. 9-2 to 9-5). This evaluation may help in planning therapy and in choosing patients who can benefit from synovectomy. Fourth, when there is involvement of both the shoulder and the cervical spine, a trial injection of lidocaine and Depo-Medrol (methylprednisolone acetate) can help identify the source of shoulder pain. Fifth, the arthrogram can demonstrate the loose bodies that can result in sudden exacerbation of pain. Last, the contrast study can differentiate between the various causes of a juxta-articular soft tissue mass. The differential possibilities include a dissecting cyst (Fig. 9-5), abscess cavities (Fig. 9-6), erosion of the rotator cuff with expansion of the subacromial-subdeltoid bursa (Fig. 9-6), or infiltration of the capsule and extracapsular soft tissues by such substances as amyloid.

In all types of inflammatory arthritis, the contrast-coated capsular outline is corrugated and

152

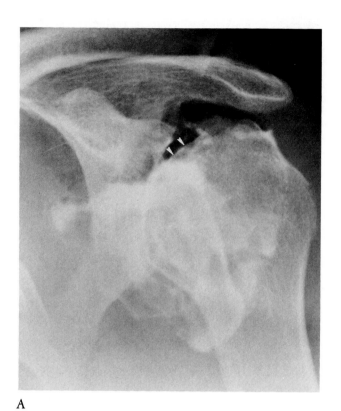

A

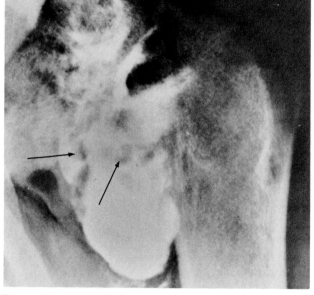

B

FIGURE 9-1. *Tuberculous arthritis.*

A, B. Internal and external rotation views of an ar-
thr>ogram demonstrate large intrasynovial-filling
defects (black arrows), loss of the smooth articular cartilage (white arrowheads), a destroyed
rotator cuff, and lymphatic drainage in the axilla.

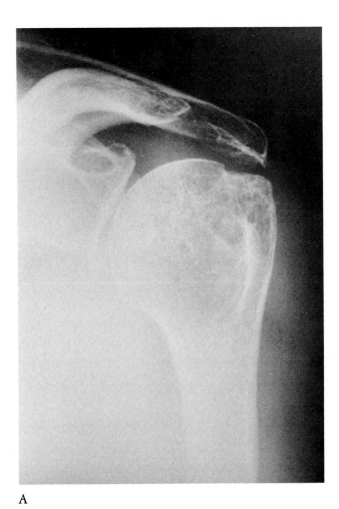

A

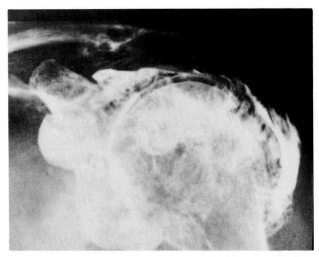

B

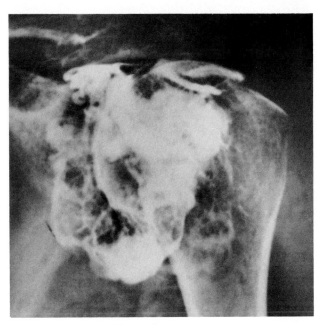

C

FIGURE 9-2. *Rheumatoid arthritis.*

A. Plain films demonstrate a normal glenohumeral joint.

B, C. Internal and external rotation views of a double contrast arthrogram show scalloping of the capsular margin, synovial hypertrophy producing irregular filling defects, and an increase in the size of the joint capsule.

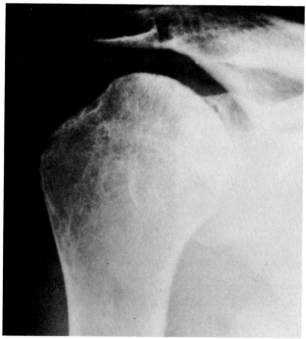

A

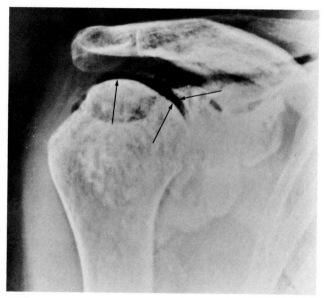

B

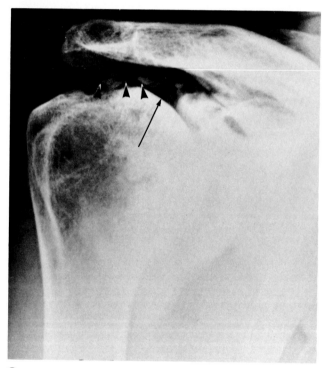

C

FIGURE 9-3. *Rheumatoid arthritis.*

  A. The plain film reveals joint space narrowing and
a high humeral head.

B, C. Internal and external rotation views of a double
contrast arthrogram demonstrate scalloping at
the capsular margin, irregular filling defects consistent with synovial hypertrophy, and almost
complete absence of the articular cartilages
(black arrows). Note that the undersurface of
the rotator cuff is eroded by pannus (black arrowheads).

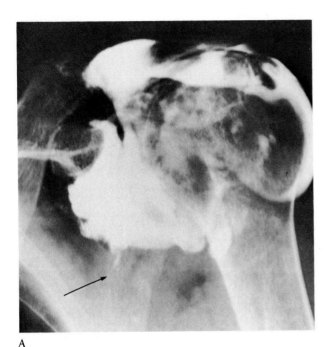

A

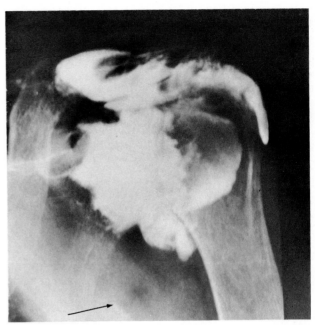

B

FIGURE 9-4. *Rheumatoid arthritis.*

A, B. Internal and external rotation views of a single contrast arthrogram reveal gross scalloping of the capsular margin, lymphatic drainage (black arrows), and complete destruction of the rotator cuff with the humeral head touching the acromion. The articular cartilages cannot be evaluated on this single contrast study.

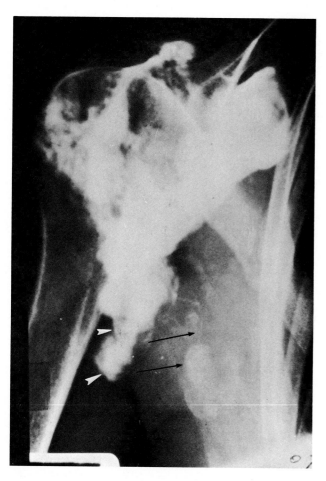

FIGURE 9-5. *Rheumatoid arthritis.*

A single contrast arthrogram demonstrates a distended irregular capsule. It contains multiple lucencies that are consistent with synovial hypertrophy. Lymphatic drainage into axillary nodes (black arrows) confirms the presence of inflammation. The axillary recess communicates with a dissecting cyst (white arrowheads).

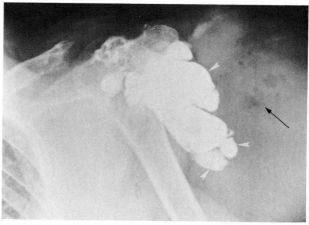

A

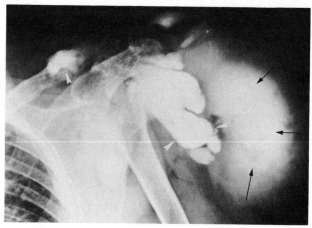

B

FIGURE 9-6. *Septic arthritis in a patient with lupus.*

A, B. The internal and external rotation views from a double contrast arthrogram demonstrate the extension of contrast into a dilated distorted sub-acromial-subdeltoid bursa (white arrowheads) and into a huge abscess cavity (black arrows) outside of the confines of the normal bursa. Lucent defects representing synovial debris are present in both cavities.

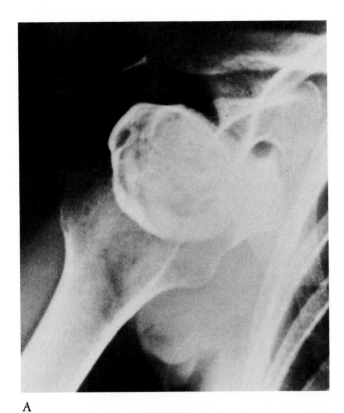

A

B

FIGURE 9-7. *Rheumatoid arthritis.*
A, B. Internal and external rotation views of a single
contrast arthrogram show a shrunken fibrotic
capsule with loss of the normal recesses and
non-filling of the biceps tendon sheath.

irregular (Figs. 9-2 to 9-5). Lymphatic drainage of contrast material can be identified and there may be filling of lymph nodes (Fig. 9-5). The articular cartilages also become narrowed and irregular (Figs. 9-2 to 9-5). Abnormal communication between the capsule and the subacromial-subdeltoid bursa can be caused by erosion of the rotator cuff by pannus (Figs. 9-3, 9-4, 9-6). If a complete tear has not yet occurred, the rotator cuff becomes narrowed and its lower margin is scalloped by inflammation from the glenohumeral joint (Fig. 9-3). Abnormal communication can also occur between the capsule and extracapsular cavities that do not correspond to a known anatomic structure (Fig. 9-6). Those cavities may represent either a dissecting synovial cyst caused by a sudden rise in intra-articular pressure (Fig. 9-5) or they may reflect the presence of an abscess associated with septic arthritis (Fig. 9-6). The proliferative arthritides (pigmented villonodular synovitis, synovial chondromatosis, and tuberculosis) produce large, distinct nodular-filling defects, reflecting synovial and subsynovial masses (see Fig. 9-1). It is important to emphasize that negative synovial fluid and a negative chest roentgenogram do not exclude tuberculous arthritis. A synovial biopsy is usually necessary to obtain an adequate culture of mycobacterium.

Long-standing inflammatory arthritis may result in contraction of the capsule with loss of the normal recesses and retraction of the insertion to the center of the humeral head (Fig. 9-7). In these cases, it may be extremely difficult to perform an intra-articular injection.

Loose Bodies

Detached osteochondral fragments can result from a variety of sources, including shoulder instability secondary to a previous dislocation, trauma, avascular necrosis, arthritis, and rarely primary synovial chondromatosis. If loose bodies are suspected, a contrast arthrogram is performed for several reasons. If an osseous or cartilaginous density is seen on the plain films, the arthrogram can differentiate between true loose bodies (Figs. 9-8, 9-9) and entities such as crystal-induced arthropathies, tumoral calcinosis, calcific tendinitis, calcific bursitis, and myositis ossificans (Fig. 9-10). If no radiopaque density is identified on the plain films and there are clinical signs of locking or crepitus, the contrast study can identify unossified loose bodies. Lastly, in the presence of a single calcified

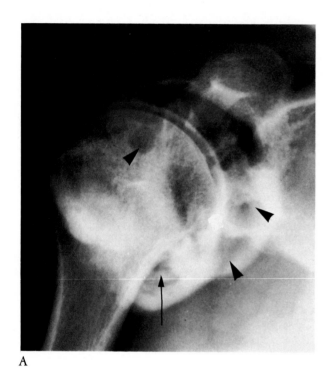

A

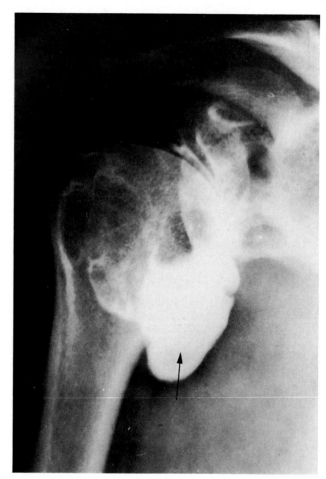

B

FIGURE 9-8. *Loose bodies.*

A, B. Internal and external rotation views of a double
contrast arthrogram show multiple round lucent
filling defects in the axillary recess (black arrowheads). Only one of these bodies was ossified
(black arrows) and visible on plain films.

Source: Goldman, A. B. Double Contrast Shoulder Arthrography. In R. H. Freiberger and J. J. Kaye (Eds.),
Arthrography. New York: Appleton-Century-Crofts,
1979.

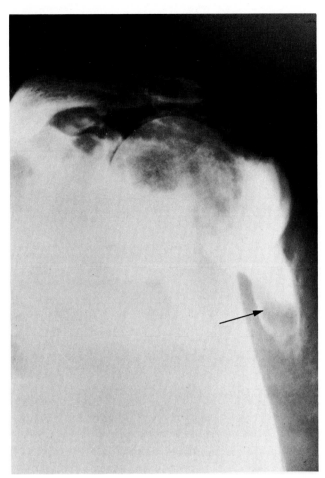

FIGURE 9-9.   *Loose bodies in biceps tendon sheath (black arrow). Plain films were negative.*

Source: Goldman, A. B. Double Contrast Shoulder Arthrography. In R. H. Freiberger and J. J. Kaye (Eds.), *Arthrography.* New York: Appleton-Century-Crofts, 1979. P. 187.

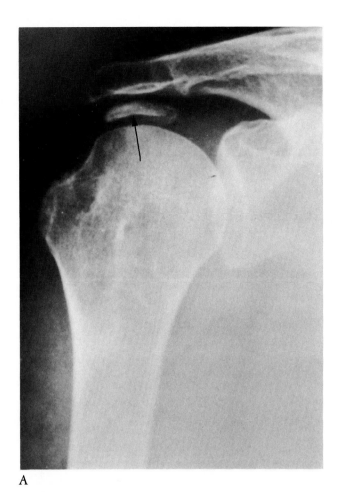

A

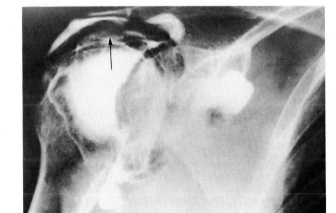

B

FIGURE 9-10.   *Myositis ossificans in a torn rotator cuff.*

A. The plain film demonstrates a density (black arrow) above the humeral head.

B. The arthrogram demonstrates the abnormal osseous fragment (black arrow) to be in the torn rotator cuff and not loose within the joint.

or ossified loose body, the arthrogram may identify other radiolucent fragments and localize their position.

If an arthrogram is performed because loose bodies are suspected, only small amounts of contrast should be used. Large amounts of positive contrast may obscure small or unmineralized fragments. In addition, multiple cross-table lateral views are often helpful in differentiating air bubbles from true loose bodies. In most instances detached osteochondral fragments migrate to the roomiest portions of the joint—the recesses. In the shoulder joint, they are most frequently identified in the axillary recess, the subscapularis bursa, and within the biceps tendon sheath. The articular portion of the shoulder joint is an extremely narrow space and it would be unusual for a fragment to lodge between the cartilaginous surfaces. In addition, an instability series should be performed on patients who have loose bodies of unknown origin to identify the site of cartilage damage.

Osteonecrosis of the Humeral Head

The disease processes that cause osteonecrosis of the humeral head are the same as those that produce this complication in the femoral head. The etiologies of osteonecrosis can be divided into four categories based on the reasons for the death of bone. The first category is trauma in which vascular compromise results from disruption of the continuity of the vessels that supply the humeral head. Neer's classification of fractures and dislocations of the shoulder emphasizes that the greater the number of displaced or angulated fragments, the greater is the likelihood of osteonecrosis [6, 8].

The second category consists of diseases that obstruct the lumen of the vessels. Sickle cell disease (abnormally shaped red blood cells) and polycythemia vera (excessive number of red blood cells) both result in clotting or sludging of the blood due to abnormalities in the cellular elements. Macroglobulinemia and heavy chain disease also increase the viscosity of the blood but affect its noncellular components. Caisson disease obstructs the lumens of vessels by nitrogen emboli and pancreatitis by fat emboli.

The third category of causes of osteonecrosis is composed of disease entities that affect the vessel wall, specifically, radiation therapy and collagen vascular diseases.

Finally, vascular supply can be compromised by processes that expand the marrow compartment of the bone and compress the vessel from the outside in. This group includes Gaucher's disease, Cushing's disease (endogenous or exogenous), and caisson disease (nitrogen diffuses into fat and increases marrow volume). In the experience at the Hospital for Special Surgery, lupus, with or without steroid therapy, was the most common reason for avascular necrosis of the humeral head.

The clinical presentation of osteonecrosis of the humeral head is often less dramatic than the clinical presentation of osteonecrosis of the femoral head. This clinical difference is probably based on the fact that the shoulder is not a weight-bearing joint, and collapse of the articular surface is frequently delayed. However, symptoms can eventually occur and cause both pain and limitation of motion. The diagnosis is usually suspected clinically because the primary disease process has already been well established by the time shoulder symptoms appear.

The plain film appearance of osteonecrosis of the humeral head is variable and depends on a balance between the severity of the vascular insult and the availability of collateral blood supply [9, 10]. In cases where irreversible damage has occurred and collapse is inevitable, a subchondral crescent fracture occurs in the humerus just as it does in the femur [5]. However, in the shoulder, the crescent involves the superior medial surface rather than the superolateral surface (Fig. 9-11). In addition, the detached cortical fragment may remain in its normal position while the subchondral bone collapses beneath it, leaving behind a "flying fragment." Increased density of the humeral head is also present and is due to a combination of the following factors: absence of normal osteoporosis (there is no blood supply to remove the mineral from the devascularized bone), compression fractures, creeping substitution, and the saponification of marrow.

If collateral blood supply has successfully compensated for the vascular damage, the plain film appearance is variable. In some cases, the humeral head preserves its normal rounded shape and a band of subchondral sclerosis, "the snow cap," parallels the superomedial aspect of the humeral head [1, 9] (Fig. 9-12A). In other patients, a round zone of lucency surrounded by a hazy sclerotic rim, "the pseudochondroblastoma," occupies the end of the

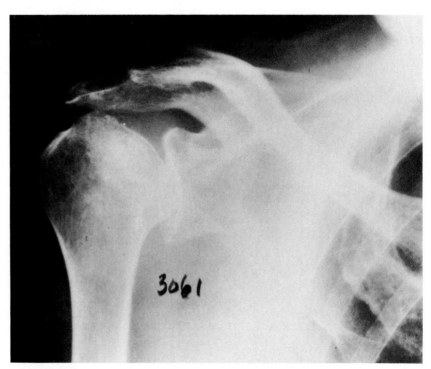

A

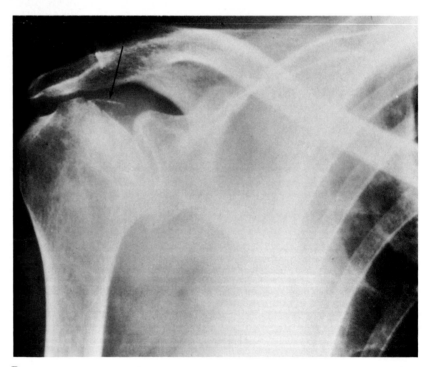

B

FIGURE 9-11. *Avascular necrosis of the humeral head.*
Internal, A, and external, B, rotation views reveal a
subchondral crescent fracture in the superomedial aspect of the humeral head. On the external rotation
view, B, the head has collapsed leaving behind a "flying
fragment" (black arrow).

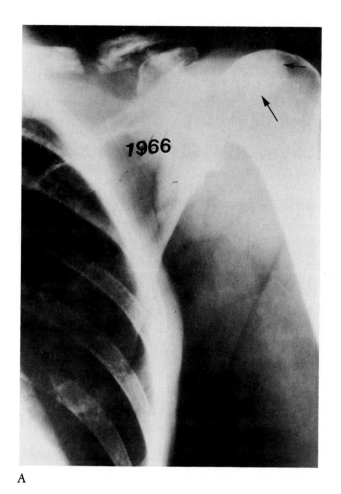

A

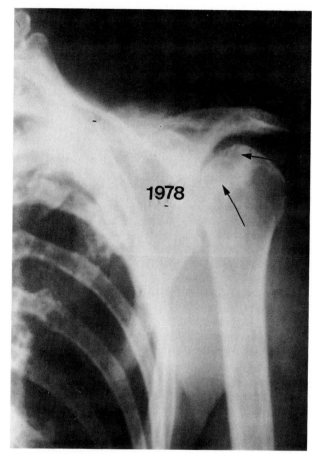

B

FIGURE 9-12. *Avascular necrosis of the humeral head secondary to radiation therapy.*

A. In 1966 the roentgenograms showed an abnormal area of sclerosis in the superomedial aspect of the humeral (black arrows). The humeral head still appears rounded. The clavicle is dense and fragmented.

B. A follow-up film, obtained in 1978, shows an area of lucency surrounded by a sclerotic rim (black arrows). There is flattening of the superomedial articular surface as well.

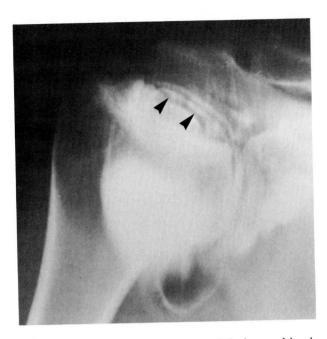

FIGURE 9-13. *Avascular necrosis of the humeral head.*
An arthrotomogram reveals air and contrast extending into the subchondral crescent fracture (black arrowheads) and outlining a loose body of dead bone.

bone [3] (Fig. 9-12B). These findings are not static, particularly in patients with systemic diseases, and the plain film abnormalities can change over a period of months [4, 5].

The role of the shoulder arthrogram in patients with osteonecrosis is not diagnostic. The diagnosis of osteonecrosis is established either by plain film findings or by radionuclide bone scan. However, the contrast study is of considerable use in the early identification of the complications of osteonecrosis, such as collapse of the articular surface or formation of loose bodies (Fig. 9-13). It can also evaluate the status of the rotator cuff and the integrity of the articular cartilages. Both of these factors can influence the choice of surgery.

If an arthrogram is to be performed on a patient with osteonecrosis of the humeral head, as little contrast as possible should be used, since excessive contrast can hide small osteochondral fragments. Tomography is also extremely helpful in these instances since the humeral head is a broad, spherical structure, and a thin line of air dissecting into a previously unidentified subchondral crescent fracture may not be readily apparent on the initial arthrographic studies (Fig. 9-13).

EVALUATION OF THE TOTAL SHOULDER REPLACEMENT

In the patient with a shoulder arthroplasty, knowledge of the etiology of pain is essential for proper treatment. The two most common reasons for the removal or replacement of a prosthesis are loosening and/or infection. The preoperative diagnosis can be established by roentgenographic technique including serial plain films, shoulder aspiration, and arthrography.

Loosening of a shoulder prosthesis can occur alone or in association with infection. They share similar plain film and arthrographic findings and can therefore be discussed together. In patients with these complications, plain film findings may or may not be present.

The plain film criteria for loosening and/or infection of a prosthesis embedded in radiopaque cement include

1. A lucent line—2 mm or wider—completely or partially surrounding the cement of one or both components
2. A horizontal fracture within the cement itself

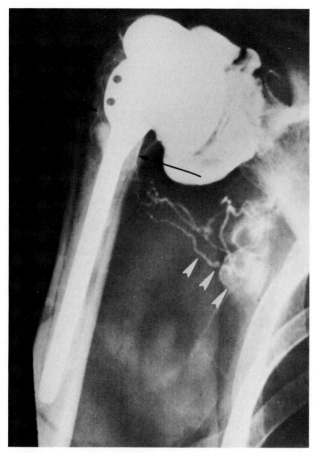

A

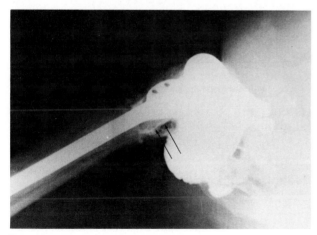

B

FIGURE 9-14. *Total shoulder replacement.*

A, B. External rotation and axillary views of a single contrast arthrogram demonstrate contrast extending into the cement bone interface of the humeral component (black arrows) indicating loosening. Lymphatic drainage (white arrowheads) does *not* mean infection—only inflammation.

3. Migration or change of alignment of the prosthesis
4. Periosteal new bone formation along the humeral shaft

Serial plain films provide the most substantial documentation of loosening, since a lucent line that increases over a period of time is more significant than one that measures greater than 2 mm. A change in the alignment of the components can only be evaluated by comparison with previous studies.

The arthrogram is performed to obtain culture material, to confirm loosening of a component when the plain films are suggestive, and to diagnose loosening of a component when the plain films are negative. The shoulder aspiration, performed on a patient with an infected prosthesis, is far less reliable than one performed on a patient with a normal shoulder joint. There are several reasons for this poor correlation. First, it is difficult to insert a needle into the fibrotic pseudocapsule. Second, in some cases, the infection becomes walled off in a pocket that does not necessarily communicate with the major portion of the pseudocapsule. Third, there is a higher incidence of anaerobic infections that are difficult to culture. If the fluid sent for culture and smear is positive, this is an excellent sign of an infected prosthesis. If, however, the culture is negative, a septic joint cannot be excluded.

The arthrographic evaluation of loosening, like the aspiration, is only helpful when it is positive. The extension of contrast material into a space between the cement and the bone (Fig. 9-14) or, less frequently, into a space between the metal and the cement indicates loosening of the component. If the initial radiographs are negative, they are repeated following exercise. False-negative studies result if loosening occurs at the distal end of the stem of the humeral component or if the interface is filled with granulation tissue and contrast material cannot reach the affected areas.

Lymphatic opacification is frequently seen in patients with infection or loosening of a prosthesis (Fig. 9-14). However, it can also be seen in patients without these complications, and therefore lymphatic opacification is not always of diagnostic significance.

Opacification of an abnormal para-articular cavity is the only arthrographic finding that indicates infection rather than loosening. Visualization of the subacromial-subdeltoid bursa—even with a prosthesis—indicates rupture of the rotator cuff, just as it does in the normal shoulder.

There is limited experience in the evaluation of total shoulder replacements, and most of these conclusions are drawn from extensive experience with total hip prostheses [2].

TREATMENT

The inflammatory arthritides, degenerative joint disease, post-traumatic arthritis, and osteonecrosis can all result in disabling pain and loss of motion in the shoulder. In all of these disorders, a course of conservative therapy is usually carried out prior to any consideration of surgery. Noninterventional treatment includes modification of daily activities, anti-inflammatory medications, physiotherapy, and in some cases corticosteroid injections. Surgery is considered only when these measures fail. In patients with systemic arthritides (e.g., rheumatoid arthritis or psoriatic arthritis), problems in the hand and elbow must be evaluated and treated first. The success of shoulder surgery strongly depends on postoperative physiotherapy, and pain in the distal joints can severely interfere with postoperative treatment.

Newer surgical techniques directed toward severe irreversible humeral head and/or glenohumeral pathology include hemiarthroplasties and total joint arthroplasties, which were popularized by Neer [7]. Hemiarthroplasty consists of the replacement of the humeral head with a conforming ball-and-stem prosthesis. Because only one side of the joint is replaced, hemiarthroplasty is primarily used in cases where the articular surface of the glenoid is not severely involved (e.g., cases with avascular necrosis of the humeral head or with a four-part fracture of the proximal humerus).

A total shoulder arthroplasty involves the replacement of both articular surfaces. Three major types of devices are now available. The first type, and type most frequently used at the Hospital for Special Surgery, is the surface replacement. The humeral side of the joint is replaced with a prosthesis similar to the Neer hemiarthroplasty, and the glenoid is covered by a polyethylene resurfacing disc that is embedded into the glenoid neck by radiopaque methyl methacrylate cement. The nonconstrained prostheses depend on an intact rotator cuff for stability. A second type is the semiconstrained prosthesis, which provides increased coverage of the humeral component by the glenoid component. It can be used in patients with defective soft tissue support, although a portion of intact rotator cuff is necessary for success. The third type is the constrained device that is designed so that the humeral and glenoid components are connected to one another. They provide stability and are recommended for patients who have severe loss of soft tissue support. The constrained devices are more susceptible to breakage and loosening.

The choice between hemiarthroplasty and total shoulder replacement depends on the integrity of the glenoid. The choice between the constrained and nonconstrained types of total shoulder arthroplasty depends on the presence or absence of soft tissue support from the rotator cuff. Therefore, the shoulder arthrogram, which can demonstrate both the glenoid labrum and the integrity of the rotator cuff, can provide important preoperative information.

REFERENCES

1. Davidson, J. K., Harrison, J. A. B., Jacobs, P., et al. The significance of bone islands, cystic areas and sclerotic areas in dysbaric osteonecrosis. *Clin. Radiol.* 28:381, 1977.
2. Dussault, R. G., Goldman, A. B., and Ghelman, B. Radiologic diagnosis of loosening and infection in hip prostheses. *J. Can. Assoc. Radiol.* 28:119, 1977.
3. Gohel, V. K., Dalinka, M. K., and Edeiken, J. Ischemic necrosis of the femoral head simulating chondroblastoma. *Radiology* 107:543, 1973.
4. Halpern, A. A. Massive synovial cyst of the shoulder causing vascular compromise. A case report. *Clin. Orthop.* 143:151, 1979.
5. Martel, W., and Poznanski, A. K. The effect of traction on the hip in osteonecrosis. A comment on the "radiolucent crescent line." *Radiology* 94:505, 1970.
6. Neer, C. S., II. Displaced proximal humeral fracture. Classification and evaluation. *J. Bone Joint Surg.* 52(A):1077, 1970.
7. Neer, C. S., II. Replacement arthroplasty for glenohumeral arthritis. *J. Bone Joint Surg.* 52(A):1, 1974.
8. Neer, C. S., II. Fractures and Dislocations of the Shoulder. In C. A. Rockwood and D. P. Green (eds.), *Fractures.* Philadelphia: Lippincott, 1975. Pp. 587, 609–610.
9. Resnick, D., and Niwayama, G. *Diagnosis of Bone*

and Joint Disorders. Philadelphia: Saunders, 1981. Pp. 2847–2851, 2858.

10. Sweet, D. E., and Madewell, J. E. Pathogeneses of Osteonecrosis. In D. Resnick and G. Niwayama (eds.), *Diagnosis of Bone and Joint Disorders with Emphasis on Articular Abnormalities.* Philadelphia: Saunders, 1981. Pp. 2780–2831.

SUGGESTED READING

Chung, S. M. K., Alavi, A., and Russell, M. O. Management of osteonecrosis in sickle-cell anemia and its genetic variants. *Clin. Orthop.* 130:158, 1978.

Coughlin, M. J., Morris, J. M., and West, W. F. Semiconstrained total shoulder arthroplasty. *J. Bone Joint Surg.* 61(A):574, 1979.

Creuss, R. L. Steroid-induced avascular necrosis of the head of the humerus. Natural history and management. *J. Bone Joint Surg.* 58(B):313, 1976.

DeSmet, A. A., Ting, Y. M., and Weiss, J. J. Shoulder arthrography in rheumatoid arthritis. *Radiology* 116:601, 1975.

Gelberman, R. H., Menon, J., Austerlitz, M. S., et al. Pyogenic arthritis of the shoulder in adults. *J. Bone Joint Surg.* 62(A):550, 1980.

Marmor, L. Hemiarthroplasty for the rheumatoid shoulder joint. *Clin. Orthop.* 122:201, 1977.

Martel, W., and Sitterley, B. H. Roentgenographic manifestations of osteonecrosis. *A.J.R.* 106:509, 1969.

Nelson, D. H. Arthrography of the shoulder joint. *Br. J. Radiol.* 25:134, 1952.

Sparbaro, J. L., Jr. The rheumatoid shoulder. *Orthop. Clin. North Am.* 6:593, 1975.

DATE DUE

NO 5 '96			